CRS

COMPUTER-RELATED SYNDROME

The Prevention
& Treatment of
Computer-Related
Injuries

RICHARD DEAN SMITH, M.D.
& STEVEN T. GARSKE, M.S., P.T.

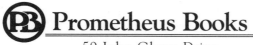 Prometheus Books

59 John Glenn Drive
Amherst, New York 14228-2197

Published 1997 by Prometheus Books

01 00 99 98 97   5 4 3 2 1

Library of Congress Cataloging-in-Publication Data

Smith, Richard Dean.
      CRS, computer-related syndrome : the prevention & treatment of computer-related injuries / Richard Dean Smith & Steven T. Garske.
            p.   cm.
      ISBN 1–57392–145–9 (paper : alk. paper)
      1. Microcomputers—Health aspects. 2. Overuse injuries. I. Garske, Steven T. II. Title.
RC965.V53S65   1997
616.9′083—dc21   97–6575
                                                                          CIP

Printed in the United States of America on acid-free paper

Contents

Acknowledgments

We wish to express our appreciation to those who have lent support and assistance to the preparation of this work, especially Adrienne Wong Hull, Cher Johnen, Maureen Fix, Heidi McGregor Garske, and Cynthia Jocson.

A special debt of gratitude is owed to Sheila Pyatt, Occupational Health Nurse for Levi Strauss, Inc., who is at the front lines every day, and in contact with all parties involved in the problems of the computer in the workplace.

Thanks are also due to Helen Reyes, Librarian, John Muir Medical Center, Walnut Creek, California, for valuable assistance and sustained interest in the project.

To literary agent Helen McGrath, we extend our sincere appreciation and gratitude.

At Prometheus Books we acknowledge the skill and expertise of Kathy Deyell.

Preface

Most writers today have converted to computers for their craft rather than pen and ink or mechanical or electric typewriters. The ease of entering text, word wrap-around, transferring blocks of text (on-screen editing), access to information, and many other features, as well as the relatively low cost, have won over most writers to the computer. These conveniences have increased productivity—the computer is faster than the unaided human hand. The usual movements of the writer or typist have been reduced to a minimum, so there is almost no need for the writer to stir from his chair for hours at a time. Numerous aids and supports that permit the writer to reduce movement even further are now available. However, the combination of increased productivity, greater focus of attention, restricted arm movement, and trunk posture have given rise to a new epidemic of computer-related complaints.

Virtually every office, home, or business has or will soon have a computer, increasing the number of individuals at risk. Yet, using a computer need not be hazardous if basic principles are followed. While much attention has been given to the hands and forearms, writers and computer workers also experience symptoms related to the upper arm, shoulders, and neck. Any prevention or treatment must take into account the entire "fore-quarter," including the entire upper extremities, neck, back, and head.

Tightness, stiffness, and pain of the upper extremities are common complaints of writers and computer users. In the early stages these complaints go unnoticed until they are so intense that the discomforts interfere with the writer's ability to write or the computer worker to work. The management teams of companies that employ a number of people who work all or most of the day at a computer keyboard seldom become aware of the workers' difficulties until the workers have experienced symptoms for long periods: weeks, months, and sometimes years.

It has been called "repetitive strain injury," "cumulative trauma disorder," "occupational cervical-brachial [neck and arm] disorders," "overuse syndromes," "work related disorders," "regional musculo-skeletal disorders," "occupational disorders of the upper extremities," and more recently, "upper extremity musculo-skeletal disorders" (UEMSD). We choose to refer to it as CRS, computer-related syndrome. The number of names for these conditions alone illustrates the confusing nature and the state of development of understanding on the prevalence and importance of these difficulties of the writer and computer keyboard worker.

The purpose of this book is to call attention to these common problems of computer use and to offer recommendations to reduce the risk of sustaining injuries related to posture, rapid movements, and positional errors common to writers and computer users. Throughout the book the terms "writer" and "computer worker" will be used interchangeably, and although we focus our attention on these occupations, the same principles apply to others at risk for injuries to the upper extremities.

Each anatomical area is treated separately, but they are not separate. What affects the hand may affect the shoulder, and vice versa. For sake of clarity, each area has been given its own special considerations.

Our intent is to cover the practical considerations that we want all computer workers to know. No book can cover every individual problem and all of the special considerations of each person. If any aspect of this book conflicts with your doctor's advice, be certain to obtain his or her approval before starting or continuing any exercise or recommendation. Above all, be aware of discomfort or symptoms and respect their importance to your ability to write.

1

The Problem

The occurrence of upper-extremity occupational repetitive injuries predates the advent of the computer by at least several centuries. As far back as 1713, Dr. Bernardino Ramazzini described pain in the hands of scribes, thus, "writer's cramp," or focal dystonia, has been known since at least the early eighteenth century. Symptoms that we now recognize as upper-extremity strain injury affected telegraphers and other manual tradesmen in the mid-nineteenth century. In Herman Melville's story "Bartleby, the Scrivener," published in 1853, one of the law copyists grinds his teeth audibly, and constantly adjusts the height of his table "for the sake of easing his back." If the table were at the wrong angle "he declared that it stopped the circulation in his arms."[1] This describes several of the problems of the modern writer at the computer keyboard. In 1897, Henry James, at age fifty-four, gave up writing and dictated to secretaries because of pain in his hand.

The Remington Arms Company developed the typewriter keyboard in 1873, but the typewriter did not immediately become a major cause of occupational injury since it required considerable effort to operate, and it could not be typed upon very rapidly. The QWERTY system key arrangement (so named because the letters on the top row of keys begin with Q, W, E, R, T, and Y) places the most commonly used keys at wide distances apart to avoid jamming the hammers of the typewriter. Old-time typists sitting at Underwood, Remington, or Royal mechanical typewriters worked with a great deal of movement of the arms and shoulders, sitting erect, frequently changing position, throwing the return lever, and adding new sheets of paper. Typing at that time was an almost aerobic exercise: Typists experienced little of the difficulty that afflicts modern writers and computer workers.

Those affected by over-use syndromes of the upper extremities are writers, musicians, and computer workers, along with grocery checkers, poultry workers, meat packers, accountants, lawyers, and many other occupations. A new industrial epidemic began with the use of electronic devices such as check-out scanners in addition to the computer. The prevalence of computers in the modern community is truly astonishing: home, school, work, music, sports —everywhere! And now, worldwide use of computers extends to some of the remotest parts of the globe.

Writers and other computer keyboard workers must be regarded as "armchair athletes" who are subject to the physical ailments of the football quarterback or baseball pitcher by developing strains and injuries to the muscles of the forearm, arm, neck, and shoulders. Repetitive strain injury, cumulative trauma disorder, and other problems of the upper extremities are mainly due to prolonged repetitive, forceful, or awkward hand movements; poor posture; "static loading" or holding a posture which promotes muscle tension for an extended period; poor conditioning of heart and lungs and poor muscle endurance; poorly fitting furniture; and the basic inadequacies of keyboard design, and are accentuated by fast-paced or heavy work loads and performance stress. The principle causes of these disorders are pressure for speed and endurance of the small muscles of the hand and forearm, as well as static postures of the trunk, neck, shoulders, and arms.

The areas most often affected are the muscles, tendons, and nerves of neck, shoulders, forearm, and hand, producing complaints of weakness, numbness, and impairment of motor control. Symptoms may also occur in the upper back, shoulder blades, and other areas of the trunk. Slow accumulation of injury occurs with gradual development of difficulty in ordinary activities, such as opening doors, holding newspapers, lifting dishes, using a hairbrush, shaking hands, or even holding a coffee cup. These symptoms may occur with or without pain and are part of the disorders associated with computer keyboard use.

The "musculotendon unit," where muscle and tendon join, is at risk: Most initial symptoms of repetitive strain injury arise from muscle and a small percent from nerve injury. When the amount of microtrauma (microscopic injury) exceeds the tissues' ability to recover, injury occurs. Microtrauma of the musculotendon unit produces inflammation and swelling of muscle and tendon fibers, which results in a reduced blood supply to the injured tissues, and eventually scarring, in which fibrous tissue forms, replacing healthy muscle tissue. The muscle disorder of repetitive strain injury appears to precede and probably leads to neurovascular entrapment, the compression of nerve tissue and blood vessels, such as carpal tunnel syndrome, a pressure on the median nerve at the wrist. Thus, the prevention of the muscle disorder repetitive strain injury is of foremost importance. Nerve entrapment may also occur in the neck, chest (the thoracic outlet syndrome), elbow (the cubital tunnel syndrome), or anywhere along the course of a nerve.

The risk of muscular disorders in keyboard workers increases if work load is increased in hours per day, or if the cumulative hours per week is increased. The pace or intensity of work further increases risk of developing repetitive strain disorder of the upper extremity, which is aggravated by poor writing habits, improper work posture, and performance stress resulting from deadlines and other realities of business life. Even though keyboard workers appear to be sedentary, they are at greater risk for physical injury than heavy industrial workers!

On average, the onset of occupational repetitive strain injury occurs at age thirty-seven in women, and forty-one in men, but it may occur at almost any age. Weakness of the arms occurs due to deconditioning* of the muscles of the neck, chest, arms, shoulder, and shoulder blade: the rotator cuff mus-

---

*Deconditioning of the muscles involves a decrease in muscle bulk, blood supply, strength, and endurance.

cles of the shoulder, pectoralis major, serratus ante-
rior, and triceps muscles. Force, along with rapid
repetition, impact stress, and awkward, static, or
strained postures are the factors which cause
upper-extremity occupational injury and other disorders of the upper extremity associated with use of
the computer keyboard.*

The computer seldom fatigues or wears out. Un-
like the typewriter, it is lightning fast, cannot jam,
and eliminates the need to strike the "return" key or
to change paper. Thus, learning how to use the computer keyboard safely becomes a major challenge.
The best and most competent workers are at the
greatest risk. The most motivated workers, those
with the highest production levels, are the ones who
tend to experience the most trouble with discomforts and problems of the upper extremities.

Disorders of the upper extremities account for 80
percent of the cost of worker's compensation. Disability claims for private insurance by doctors,
lawyers, accountants, dentists, writers, etc. for
upper-extremity disorders have increased nearly
fivefold in the past five years. By the beginning of
the twenty-first century, three-fourths of all jobs
will require computer keyboard use, placing a huge
work force at risk.[2] And the potential for harm
doesn't end there. Industry will begin to accrue additional costs—time lost from work by the injured
employees, missed deadlines, the need to hire and
train replacement workers—that at some point will
inevitably be passed along to the consumer.

The social cost of computer-related syndrome

---

*Throughout this book the term "upper extremity" will be used
to refer to the hand, wrist, arm, shoulder, and shoulder blade.

(CRS) and repetitive strain injury—the tragic personal toll of loss of self-esteem and health—equals the financial costs. Time may be lost from writing, and some writers may be unable to write, cook, garden, or pick up their children because of CRS.

NOTES

1. Herman Melville, "Bartleby, The Scrivener," in *The Piazza Tales and Other Prose Pieces, 1829–1860,* Harrison Hayford, Alma A. McDonald, and Thomas Tanselle, eds., p. 17 (Evanston and Chicago: Northwestern University Press, 1987).

2. Thomas A. Hales, "Medical Management of Upper Limb Disorders. The ANSI Experience," Paper presented at the International Conference on Occupational Disorders of the Upper Extremities, San Francisco, December 1–2, 1994.

2

What the Computer Worker Experiences

The writer or computer keyboard user is at risk for CRS, repetitive strain injury, or other problems of the upper extremities if she uses the computer two or more hours a day. Some individuals may work much longer without symptoms, but two hours per day over a period of time increases the risk of developing injuries related to computer use.

Symptoms of CRS depend on what area of the upper extremity is involved. The principal tissue areas that cause difficulties are muscle and tendon. The "musculotendinous junction," the area where the tendon and muscle join, is particularly vulnerable to this type of injury. Although such a junction occurs at each end of the muscle, the "distal" end, that which is farthest from the center of the body, is most at risk. Studies of actual anatomical sites of the upper extremity are limited because the condi-

19

tion is not such that extensive (biopsy or pathological) studies have been carried out.

The most common complaint and the earliest symptom is a sensation of *tightness* of the hands, wrists, or the muscles of the forearm between the wrist and elbow. Initially, tightness tends to develop after a period of writing and lasts longer with continued use. Tightness is often accompanied by loss of flexibility of the joints operated by the particular muscles. In the case of the forearm, the wrist may not have its usual ability for full flexion (bending) or extension (straightening). Such movements may feel comfortable within a limited range, but at the extremes of the joint's normal range, a sensation of tightness and pulling is noted and may be accompanied by a feeling of soreness.

The writer may note *tenderness* of specific areas of the upper extremity, especially tenderness of the muscles of the forearm, upper arm, and shoulder, and the muscles of the neck. Tenderness over other localized sites, such as the heel of the hands and the bony prominences of the elbows, also occurs and will be discussed in the following sections.

A sensation of *pain* in muscle areas of the upper extremity is very common. Initially, pain occurs after an extended period at the computer, but as CRS advances, the pain occurs with progressively shorter periods of use to the point that the writer may not be able to perform his or her usual or necessary writing tasks without pain. In the case of more severe injury, the individual continues to experience pain away from writing. In the most debilitating instances of injury, the pain persists and disturbs the person's rest and sleep. The pain varies from a deep aching, pulling soreness, to a sharp, tearing feeling.

In many instances, the fingers, hands, and fore-arms may feel swollen and tight. *Swelling* may not be apparent to an observer, but the use of muscles increases blood flow to that area with dilation of blood vessels leading to edema (swelling) or a tiny amount of fluid collection in the spaces outside the blood vessels and muscles. The swelling occurs in a confined space, which leads to resistance of blood flow to muscle and tendinous tissues, resulting in relative "ischemia," or insufficient blood supply. Reduced blood circulation provides an inadequate supply of oxygen and slows the removal of metabolic waste products. If the muscle areas are repeatedly subjected to ischemia due to excessive use, the muscles become shortened and more subject to microtrauma. Excessive stretching of the muscle fibers results in scarring and further reduction of blood flow, which leads to noxious substances being trapped within the muscle.

If the muscles become swollen and enlarged in a confined space, pressure on the nerve of the area, especially the forearm, occurs, leading to compression of neural tissue. This may cause symptoms of *numbness* and tingling, decreased sensation, and weakness—either a decrease or loss of sensation in the fingers and hands, or a disturbance in sensation such as burning, crawling, electric, buzzing, pinching, or other uncomfortable feelings.

The symptoms of upper-extremity injury slowly increase, or they may be intermittent for a considerable period of time. In some instances, the discomfort of the hands and arms is persistent from the onset. Occasionally, a precipitous overload of the arms and hands either due to excessive use or to a new or more strenuous activity may precipitate a sudden cascade of symptoms.

As the changes in the muscle and tendinous tissues due to injury accumulate, tolerance for writing gradually decreases. This is evident in the decreasing amount of time the writer can use the keyboard before symptoms appear. The condition may degenerate to the point that the writer can hardly touch the keyboard, raise a glass, lift a baby, or shake hands.

Continued use of the hands and arms after the writer experiences symptoms increases the risk of permanent injury. Either by the severity of the pain or intolerance to the activity of writing, the individual may be forced to give up use of the hands entirely.

When observed, the computer worker often exhibits hazardous postures and harmful techniques at the keyboard. One difficulty leads to another, and one small area of distress can spread to other areas, since improper use of the hands also leads to problems with the arms and shoulders and neck. The computer worker often experiences muscular tightness of the arms, shoulders, and neck. Pain and weakness lead to development of abnormal movement patterns. Even the jaw, or temporomandibular joint, plays a part in the development of distress, potential limitations, and disability of the computer worker.

Who is at risk? Although some writers can work long periods at the keyboard without experiencing these problems, no one is free from the risk of computer-related syndrome. Nevertheless, those who work hardest are at the greatest risk for occupational disorders of the upper extremity. Highly motivated individuals put in longer hours, work under more pressure, tend to focus on the task at hand,

and tend to ignore symptoms until they are unable to continue due to pain, loss of sensation, weakness, or loss of coordination.

The following photograph illustrates a variety of harmful postures and positions: The head is held awkwardly to the side; the shoulder is elevated and thrust forward to hold the telephone; posture is slumped and spine flexed; elbows are held out to the side, causing static loading of shoulder muscles; trunk and neck are rotated; and the list goes on.

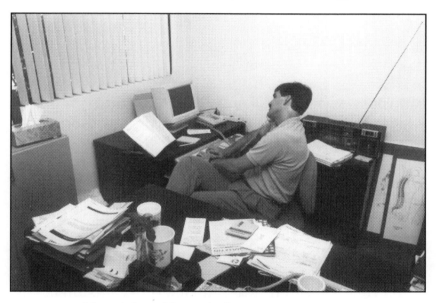

Harmful positions: A disaster in progress.

3

Clinical:
What Is Found on Examination

"Those who do not feel pain seldom think that it is felt."

Samuel Johnson, *The Rambler*

A physical examination after CRS symptoms have become too painful to ignore usually reveals little. The lack of "objective" findings is frustrating to both the writer and the examiner. In fact, usually the finding will be simply that there is a reduction of the normal *range of motion* due to muscle shortening resulting in limited flexion or extension of the wrist and fingers, shoulder motions, and motions of the neck.

Associated feelings of numbness, tingling, or crawling sensations of the arms, forearms, hands, and fingers which often do not follow the usual sensory patterns of nerves may also be complained of. The discomfort may be located in the neck; the trapezius areas above the crest of the shoulders; the shoulders; elbows; forearms; top and/or underside of the wrists; the soft, fleshy part of the palms or the center of the palms; the top of the thumbs; and the fingers, yet the examiner finds little to account for these complaints except the reaction of the writer to pressure or movement of the joints and soft tissues. *Decreased sensation* on testing with a sharp pin or touch with a loose cotton tip may be present, but may also be inconsistent with normal anatomical nerve patterns.

The writer may experience *skin-fold tenderness,* a pain or burning sensation felt when the normal loose skin fold, especially of the neck, shoulders, and forearms, is grasped and rolled gently. This may cause the patient to do more than wince; he may nearly drop to his knees from the intensity of the pain. The *skin* may show a mottled appearance over the forearms and hands. This results from vasoconstriction of the blood vessels in the skin and is not specific to keyboard-related disorders.

Although the sensation of *swelling* in the fingers, wrists, and forearms may be present, an examination often provides few objective findings to substantiate the writer's complaints of discomfort and pain. Although rings and jewelry feel tight, measurable swelling may not be detectable.

Tender areas of muscle and tendon sites tend to be similarly located in persons with computer-related syndrome. Certain trigger points in muscles, especially of the neck and shoulders, occur with consistent regularity.

To the dismay of both doctor and patient, *laboratory tests* often disclose no abnormality. General tests and occasionally a chest X-ray are sometimes performed to exclude other or associated causes of symptoms.

X-rays of the afflicted areas show few, if any, findings or abnormalities except occasionally osteoarthritis ("wear and tear" arthritis) of the fingers or spine, a common finding with or without CRS symptoms, depending in part on the patient's age and history of injury. Rarely, abnormalities within the chest may accompany symptoms of the neck and shoulders. In rare instances irritation of the diaphragm caused by inflammation in the chest or abdominal cavities may be a cause of shoulder pain. The CT scan or MRI* occasionally may show abnormalities of the spine that may or may not be related to computer use, such as an extra or "cervical" rib. Electromyograms (EMG), an electrical test of muscle and nerve function, may be abnormal in certain cases of nerve entrapments, such as carpal tunnel syndrome.

Other than tenderness of characteristic areas, limitation of motion of certain joints due to muscle shortening, skin-fold tenderness, and sometimes findings on X-ray or EMG, the physical and laboratory examination provides few strictly objective findings that might convince the skeptical observer of the presence of injury.

---

*A CT scan, or computerized axial tomography, involves the gathering of anatomical information in which an X-ray scanner makes many sweeps of the body and the results are processed by computer to give a cross-sectional image. An MRI, or magnetic resonance imaging, is a diagnostic technique in which the patient's body is placed in a nuclear magnetic field and its nuclei (hydrogen) are excited by radio-frequency pulses; resulting signals are processed through a computer to produce an image.

PAIN

> Pain has an Element of Blank;
> It cannot recollect
> When it began, or if there were
> A time when it was not.
>
> It has no future but itself.
> Its infinite realms contain
> Its past, enlightened to perceive
> New periods of pain.
>
> > Emily Dickinson,
> > "Pain Has an Element of Blank"

Pain is the most common complaint that causes the writer or computer worker to seek medical attention. Since tendons and joint capsules (the tissue supporting the joint) are richly supplied with pain fibers (nerve endings), what is actually microscopic physical injury may be interpreted by the brain as intensely painful because many pain fibers are activated. Muscle tissue also contains pain fibers, but they are less concentrated. Such a disturbance may be interpreted by the individual as intense pain if located in an area rich in pain fibers, such as the neck, shoulder, palm, and fingers. Pain is an adaptive symptom of injury, a warning calling the individual to take precautions.

Treatments for pain vary from minor medicines to major interventions based on extent and cause. Few medicines are recommended in early treatment of CRS. As long as the writer continues to participate in the activities that brought on and aggravate the injury, no analgesic or pain medicine is likely to be very effective. Changing habits, posture, and use of the hands and upper extremities is much more important. In many instances, the use of analgesic medicines to permit the writer or keyboard worker to "keep going" aggravates the original problem of musculotendinous injury because the writer continues to accumulate additional injury.

As the pain persists, if the writer continues the habits and postures that cause injury, the pain may greatly accelerate and become virtually undiagnosable except as an entity called "chronic pain." In the case of chronic pain, the usual treatments are no longer effective. Every effort must be undertaken to control problems related to computer use before chronic pain occurs.

4

Prevention

"A man who suffers before it is necessary, suffers more than is necessary."

Seneca, *Letters to Lucilius*

Prevention is by far the most important consideration of the computer worker and writer. Most injuries can be prevented or minimized by knowing the risks of using the computer keyboard and practicing the basic measures useful in lessening the repetitive and static loading of the upper extremities.

Many strategies and modifications that can make an immediate difference can be undertaken easily, often with minimal or no expense. To achieve maximum success, every individual takes responsibility to monitor himself and intervene before the *symptom threshold* is exceeded. "Symptom threshold" means the point in time during an activity (or the range of motion of a movement) at which continuing the activity or movement will cause a cascade of events leading to increasing symptoms and limited ability to perform computer keyboard work. Understanding the importance of the "symptom threshold" concept is critical to the prevention of injury, because once it is passed, the symptoms can be severe and persist for hours to days. Once the symptom threshold has been exceeded, appropriate medical intervention or treatment becomes less effective.

Awareness of risk is the most important part of prevention. At risk are those who write or work at the keyboard two or more hours per day. Sitting posture and arm and hand positioning are of paramount importance. "Head back/chin down" with a neutral spine position (i.e., a balanced posture in which the normal curves of the spine are maintained), and shoulders held back and down becomes the foundation of proper posture and technique.

Rather than immobilizing hands and wrists on a wrist rest in front of the keyboard, a "high wrist" position with the wrists free and elevated above the keyboard is much more natural and easier to maintain. Curving the fingers and using the ends or tips of the fingers, not the finger pads, allows movement with less strain on the hands and fingers. Use a mirror or a buddy to check positioning of the wrist and hands to avoid awkward positioning and movements. The mirror allows the worker to monitor himself for exaggerated, awkward positions (such as forced extension of the thumb or little finger) that may otherwise go unnoticed. In an abnormal position, such as with the wrists firmly on a wrist rest, the fingers may "jump" when typing, increasing the muscle tension in the hand and forearm.

Forced extension of the little finger to get it out

of the way adds opposing muscle activity within the hand and forearm. In the same way, an extended or abducted thumb (one held away and raised) not ordinarily put to use in keyboard operation (usually the left thumb), causes tension and extra effort of the other fingers.

ADDITIONAL FACTORS TO CONSIDER

"No man can see all with his own eyes or do all with his own hands."

Samuel Johnson, *The Idler*

Watching television has the same hazards for the writer as the computer screen. Take care of your eyes, with range-of-motion movements of the eyes, changing gaze from near to far, up and down, and side to side. Look at an imaginary "H": center gaze at the middle of the crossbar; look to the left where the crossbar meets the upright bar; then up to the top of the upright; then down to the bottom of the upright bar; back to the center of the upright bar where it meets the crossbar; back to the middle of the crossbar and center vision, and repeat on the right. These actions relieve static fatigue of the eyes.

The writer's glasses may need to be adjusted or a separate pair suitable to the moderately close work at the computer may need to be obtained.

Dryness of the eyes may be caused by staring at the computer screen and infrequent blinking, and may be worsened by air conditioning and contact lenses. Relief from static positioning at the keyboard and fixed gaze on the computer screen requires interruption for the eyes as well as the arms and hands. Use eye drops (artificial tears) as necessary if the eyes continue to feel dry. If discomfort persists, have the eyes examined by an ophthalmologist. Dry eyes and eye strain may also contribute to headache and muscle tightness of the neck and shoulders.

Since most writers are avid readers, posture while reading is equally important. Lying on your stomach, propped up on your elbows, leads to static muscle tension of the neck and shoulders. Even holding a book may lead to muscle fatigue and other symptoms of the entire upper extremity. Reasonable sitting posture and something as simple as a pillow on your lap to support the weight of the book can serve to relieve much of the static muscle fatigue of the arms and hands.

The focus throughout this book is on the mature writer, but children and teenagers using the computer keyboard or video games are at risk for the same problems and disabilities. With the rise of the use of the computer keyboard and the emphasis on rapid, repetitive motions in playing video games, our young population risks injury before they are old enough to enter the job market. Simple methods and readily available materials stressed in this volume are meant to ward off this growing epidemic.

Many computer workers are on the telephone for hours each day. In addition to the physical and postural hazards of the telephone, many clients or customers are difficult or abusive. The computer worker many try to remain calm, but the physiology of the body is one of being under attack. In this circumstance, the muscles of the neck, shoulders, and back automatically become tense and frozen. Counseling the computer worker to refrain from making the client's problem his own problem, while still handling the client tactfully, is essential to the worker's own well-being as well as the company's success.

Social environment plays an important role in the development and course of disorders of the upper extremity. Musculoskeletal problems of the upper extremities are more common and more severe in workers where the demands on them are high but they have little control over their work or environment. When aggravated by monotony and lack of a feeling of self-worth, workers are more likely to perceive pressure to perform and are more sensitive to time pressure. Fear of losing a job or being replaced is a major factor in both the occurrence of upper-extremity disorders and under-reporting of symptoms. Surveillance or merely imagined surveillance increases fear, tension, and stress even when away from the workplace. The only social intervention that shows a definite effect on reducing the rate of injury is for management to understand and be aware of risks to workers and to encourage early treatment. Job dissatisfaction often relates to an increase in complaints of the upper extremities.

An individual worker with computer-related syndrome shifts more work on to the other workers, who may give the injured worker a hard time, accusing him of falling down on the job. Subsequently, when a worker begins to experience musculoskeletal discomforts, he tends to ignore or cover up the problem so as not to burden other workers. This compounds the problem, resulting in more severely injured workers who require even longer periods of time to recover. A supportive work environment and management aware of the risks to the computer worker is essential. In the long run, by recognizing

CRS and treating it early, the worker and the work unit become more productive with less time lost and more rapid recovery of injured workers.

Writers who work independently may be even more liable to push themselves far past the time when symptoms tell them to change their ways or stop writing. The writer responds to internal demands that may be even more demanding or insensitive than the worst of business management. While Shakespeare's admonition "rest a while and run a mile" may not be quite apt for the writer, the general principle applies to both the computer worker and the writer. The sooner the writer attends to herself, the sooner she will be able to write or return to writing safely and comfortably. The treatment and prevention of computer-related syndrome is a twenty-four-hours-a-day, seven-days-a-week mission.

By all means, the control of fatigue with adequate bedrest and sleep helps with general health and the ability to maintain good posture at the keyboard. To paraphrase Montaigne, "a fatigued, exhausted writer seldom produces anything to purpose." Organize time to reduce the pressure of deadlines, spend time planning your work, write smarter. Use your brain instead of relying on the muscles of your neck and arms to perform extra and unnecessary duty. Writing tends to be a labor-intensive undertaking, so try to work more efficiently without inhibiting creativity. The computer, with its ease of editing, entices the writer into careless, untidy habits of throwing ideas into the computer to sort them out on screen later. More experienced writers learn to prepare ahead, to outline, at least mentally, to have their thesis in mind before beginning the actual task of entering their work on the keyboard. By pre-writing, the writer is more effective and saves unnecessary physical stress, especially of the neck, shoulders, and arms.

BEFORE BEGINNING TO WRITE

- Warm the hands and forearms in gloves or under warm water until they are comfortably warm. This improves blood supply and reduces muscle tightness.

- Improve sitting posture by rolling the pelvis forward and back, then stop at the midpoint.

- Stretch the arms, hands, shoulder, and neck muscles as described in chapters 14 and 15.

- Learn to relax the arms and hands even when intent on your task.

- Avoid abnormal and uncomfortable postures that increase muscle tension and cause extra effort.

DURING WORK

- Take regular breaks away from the keyboard. In the long run, the writer will be more productive if measures that reduce the demands on the upper extremities and the neck are followed.

- Check posture and position of hands and arms frequently until a desirable position and posture becomes natural.

- Instead of resting the forearms on an arm rest or the wrists on a wrist pad, maintain a *floating arms* position where the arms and hands float above the keyboard with a natural motion. The best arm position can be better achieved by the *elbow flap*—holding the arms out from the sides of the chest and allowing them to "flap" against the sides of the chest several times. This relaxes the muscles of the arms and shoulders, allowing the arms to hang naturally and avoiding the static loading of the shoulder muscles caused by holding the arms away from the body.

- Change position. Stand up and stretch long before you think you need to. Raise your arms over head and gently wiggle fingers to lessen swelling and static positioning.

- Use deep and proper abdominal/diaphragmatic breathing to help maintain a relaxed attitude and lessen the effort of the confinement of writing and keyboard work.

- Use relaxation techniques to lessen the strain and wear on the muscle and tendons of the hands and forearms.

5

The Workstation

"We put our love where we have put our labor."
Ralph Waldo Emerson, *Journals*

Although much effort has been directed toward making the workstation more efficient, efficient design has resulted in a new problem—workstations are *too* good, *too* efficient! With new designs, everything the writer or computer worker needs is close at hand. The writer has so many conveniences that little effort is expended in movements such as reaching for a disk or the printer switch. The old fashioned work-table with books on the other side of the room (which required the writer to get up from her chair to go to the reference materials) is all but gone. The new, efficient designs do not allow for enough occasions to stir the writer out of her chair, which contributes to static loading, poor conditioning, poor posture, and poor muscle tone. Everything about the workstation is designed to eliminate motion, leading to static, immobile positions that are unfavorable for the writer's overall performance.

Even the *chairs* are now designed to eliminate movement—including gravity support of the forearms. However, the chair ought *not* have arm rests, especially if they inhibit normal movement. Often the chair back is too low and the upper edge of the back causes localized pressure to the mid-back. The optimum chair design supports the mid, low, and upper back in a neutral, normal position. Many chairs supposedly designed for the writer are now adjustable to make adequate back support possible. A comfortably padded stool, such as a good piano stool, with no arm supports or back support is more desirable than a poor chair. In the best designs, the chair seat is tilted slightly forward, or has the option for an adjustable forward tilt of the chair or for the placement of a forward-tilting a seat pad.

One of the most neglected aspects of the chair is the proper *height,* which should be adjustable. The thighs should be almost parallel to the floor such that the hips are slightly higher than the knees.

Foot rests are not recommended, especially if they encourage the writer to slump back in the chair. The writer bears some weight on the feet when sitting in an optimal position. The feet are placed directly under the knees in a position allowing weight to rest on the full length of the foot rather than on the heels or toes. Avoid slumping into the back of the chair with little weight on the feet; this contributes to poor posture of the trunk, neck, and shoulders.

The computer *monitor* position may also be a problem. One example of this is the individual who had the monitor behind him, requiring long periods of sharply twisting the head and spine fully to the rear, straining the back, neck, and shoulders. In a correct position, the monitor is placed close enough so the writer does not have to lean forward or strain to read the screen, and is at a level so the writer does not need to look up or down.

Usually the top edge of the monitor should be positioned at eye level, not at a height where eye level is at the center of the screen. The font size in most programs is easily changed to one large enough so that it is easy to read and to edit. The type of font also makes a great difference to the writer. While Times is a popular font for printing, it is not one that is easy to read or edit on the monitor. Courier is one of the easiest to read and edit on-screen. The elaborate typefaces are best avoided while writing, and can be changed prior to printing if a special font is desired.

The *keyboard position* is one of the most neglected features of proper keyboard technique. The keyboard position just above the thighs is optimal so that the forearms are parallel to the thighs and to the floor, with the wrists at the same height from the floor as the elbows or slightly lower, *never* higher. The following photograph demonstrates how optimal height of the keyboard allows for proper wrist and finger position while still maintaining neutral spine and shoulder positions. Use of a wrist rest that requires the fingers alone to reach excessively for out-of-the-way keys must be avoided.

The type of keyboard is of less importance than proper positioning, with a few exceptions. Usually, the best position for the keyboard is flat rather than tilted up like the old typewriters. This prevents ex-

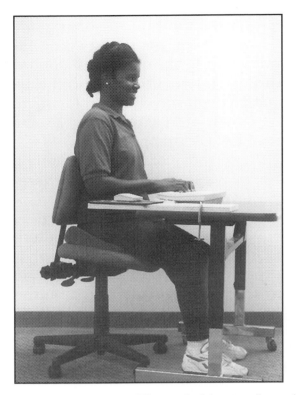

Keyboard flat and not tilted up. Elbows held naturally and nearly directly below the shoulders. Seat tilted slightly downward 15 to 20 degrees or use a "seat wedge." Hips are the same height or slightly higher than the knees. Although not pictured here, the computer monitor should be positioned so the top of it is at eye level.

cessive bending of the wrist. Place a small block or the wrist rest *under* the near edge of the keyboard so the keyboard is flat or at a slight negative tilt (i.e., it tilts away from your body).

Key pressure or resistance in keyboards may play an important role in preventing CRS. A very soft keyboard may allow the writer to hit "bottom" with each stroke, which is like striking the ends of the fingers on a hard surface thousands of times each

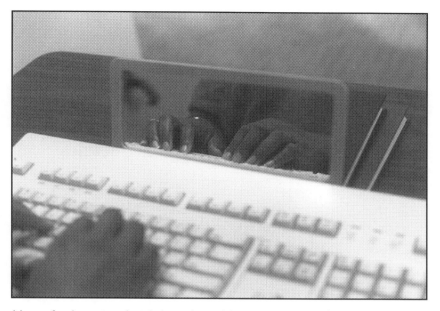

Use of mirror to check hand position and movements of fingers.

day. Writers who have a heavy stroke are better off with a higher-resistance keyboard. Even those with a soft touch are probably better off with a higher-resistance keyboard so that padding will prevent bottoming out and subsequent impact injury to the fingers and fingertips. The resistance of the keys, however, need not be so high that it encourages an even more forceful keystroke.

When the writer is concentrating intently on a writing project, the *trunk, hand, and arm postures* may fall into poor positions. Placing a small mirror in front of the keyboard allows the writer to check hand and wrist position easily and frequently without much effort (see photo above). Another way to make sure the hand and arm positions are maintained is to enlist the aid of an associate to observe and to make corrections. Although a buddy gives the writer feedback on technique which may suffice for a short time, one is not likely to be helpful over an extended period. A person simply is not capable of observing effectively for long, and the worker is at risk at all times. For those with a video recorder, videotaping the writer at work can effectively check hand position; although it may be cumbersome for the writer, it can be valuable for the therapist and physician to point out undesirable and hazardous positions and movements which have been acquired. Of the methods available, use of a small mirror is the least intrusive and most practical.

Many writers and computer workers sit at the computer for hours at a time without moving and only stir when some body part is so uncomfortable that it screams for relief. Such postures lead to *static loading* of muscles and tendinous tissues that can be relieved only by movement. Any posture that is held constant for long periods will become painful—even lying in bed. In this instance, our body parts have more sense than our brains. Here are a few suggestions that help to relieve the pain of immobility and static loading:

- Place something that is used regularly (a reference book, for example) in some other part of the house, apartment, or office, thus requiring getting up, stretching, and walking to an area *away* from the workstation.

- Do not put coffee or water in a thermos at the desk, but place it so that getting it requires movement.

- Position the printer at a distance requiring movement to use it.

- Place refills of paper or other materials in a closet out of your reach.

- Reaching for an object and hitting the end-range of the joints (e.g., fully straightening the elbow) creates more stress on the muscles, tendons, joints, and nerves of the arm. Repetitive end-range motion reaching leads to injury, pain, inflammation, and loss of motion. The farther the reach, the more stress on supporting structures, especially if the object is moderately heavy or held far away from the body. Use a *step-and-weight shift* strategy toward the object: bend at the hips, or get out of the chair to use the same reaching techniques from a standing position.

- Adjust the writing station to require the writer to move. Get up, stretch, walk around. In the process, some of the clutter of the writing trade can be cleaned away.

For those who frequently use the *telephone* during their work, such as for research or interviews, an *effective* extension on the handset that allows it to be cradled by the shoulder without side bending (lateral flexion) of the neck is preferred to reduce muscle tightness and muscle fatigue pain. Crooking the neck sideways to hold the telephone receiver is an easy, hazardous habit to acquire, but not always easy to break. If the telephone is used for long periods, a headset is preferred.

The writer's surroundings make the difference between a comfortable, pleasant place to spend one's creative life and a dreary, disheartening place that begs for relief. The workstation becomes a second home. A few friendly concessions to the environment are usually within the control of the writer. Whether at home or at the office, using proper *lighting* with enough variation and contrast relieves the monotony of the work area. Avoiding glare is essential and can be controlled by placement of the computer screen so that outside sunlight and reflection do not cause squinting or eye strain. Enough lighting and color contrast makes the environment pleasant and interesting.

To reduce glare:

- Adjust the brightness and contrast of the computer screen according to light conditions. Also, use somewhat less lighting in the room for computer work and more for paper work. Avoid white walls and desks to reduce reflection.

- Position the screen at a ninety-degree angle to a source of natural sunlight. Natural light is best not placed in front of or directly behind the monitor screen.

- Wear dark clothing to reduce glare and reflection.

- Keep the monitor screen clean and free of smudges and dirt to reduce eye strain.

- Format characters so they are large enough to read without straining, and choose colors for the background and characters that contrast enough so they are easy to read. This will also help to avoid eye strain.

Equally important for avoiding CRS is the amount of ambient *noise* surrounding the workstation. Loud, harsh, or irritating levels or quality of noise can usually be controlled to a reasonable level. The effort of concentration required to exclude noise increases tension in the muscles of the face, neck, and shoulders. Make every attempt to limit distractions. The more the writer must focus attention on excluding interfering noise, the more effort required to write. The better the control of interfering noise, the better concentration and productivity with fewer errors. Some writers find that a certain level of noise is desirable because it may enhance their ability to concentrate, but if excessive, noise becomes an obstacle to writing. A little music may make for lighter work and less monotony of chores, but may interfere with serious writing. Silence seems to terrify modern man, but quiet invites the muse of composition.

6

The Fingers Do the Walking

"When God finished speaking with Moses on
Mount Sinai, he gave him the two tablets of the
covenant, tablets of stone, written with the finger
of God."

Exodus 31:18

The role of fingers in the act of creativity is self-ev-
ident and is exquisitely expressed by Michelangelo
in the *Creation of Man,* the central fresco of the
ceiling of the Sistine Chapel. The outstretched
index finger of God reaches toward that of Adam in
one of the most compelling figures in the history of
art. The symbolism of fingers is found in many con-
texts and cultures, from the Bible quote cited above
to the "Rubaiyat of Omar Khayyam," a poem
written in a typical Middle Eastern format:

The Moving Finger writes; and having writ,
Moves on; nor all your Piety nor Wit
    Shall lure it back to cancel half a Line
Nor all your Tears wash out a single Word of it.

Because the writer or computer worker sits at a desk and makes few if any vigorous movements, the act of writing appears to the onlooker to be sedentary: Little effort is expended and there appears to be little risk of physical injury. However, as was mentioned earlier, computer workers are "armchair athletes," in that they perform athletic feats with their fingers and arms. This athletic activity of the fingers while using the computer keyboard is akin to the rapid, forceful movements of sprinters or tennis players—and no one doubts their actions are athletic, difficult, and demanding. The daily cumulative load performed by the fingers of a computer worker may amount to several tons, and is even greater in faster typists, who tend to exert higher force on keys than slower typists.

Complaints of soreness of the joints of the fingers, especially the middle joints of each finger (the proximal interphalangeal joint), and, to a lesser extent, the end joints (the distal interphalangeal joints), may occur after long use. Hard use of the fingers and continuous impact may lead in part to the development of cartilage breakdown or osteoarthritis of these finger joints.

When CRS has struck, the fingers may feel stiff and tight, with a sensation of being swollen and puffy. Although the fingers may appear normal to an observer, rings may be more difficult to get off because of slight, diffuse swelling. Clenching the hand into a fist may be difficult or even impossible at times due to swelling of many small tissues. The fingers may also feel fatigued, and they may become clumsy and less dexterous, leading to more typing mistakes, and requiring greater time and effort.

On *examination,* the fingers appear normal or show a slight diffuse swelling that cannot be readily measured by any ordinary clinical test. Although tightness of rings occurs, this is not a very accurate measurement for such small degrees of swelling. The soft tissue of the fingers may be tender or sensitive to touch, or the joints may be tender. Overt swelling and inflammation may occur, but in most instances, physical examination of the fingers demonstrates little that may be consistent with a distinct finding of physical abnormality.

CAUSE

Pinching and handling paper puts more stress on the small joints of the fingers than grasping or holding. The hand was originally "designed" to grasp and swing from trees and vines, not to handle small items. Rapid movement and long sessions at the keyboard lead to increased blood flow and dilation of blood vessels, causing edema or swelling of the small structures of the fingers. These structures are confined in tight fibrous compartments, so blood flow to the area is reduced. Poor trunk and shoulder posture leads to poor hand position, compounding the problem of the fingers.

Keyboard "bottoming" or striking the bottom of the keyboard resistance by use of a light-touch keyboard may take away some muscle stress to the forearms, but, as has been discussed, striking the ends of the fingers on a hard surface thousands of times each day can also cause discomfort.

Long fingernails are an additional hazard to the writer because they cause the writer to extend the fingers, keeping them straight so as to type with the finger pads. A more natural position allows the fingers to curve and typing to be done with the ends or tips of the fingers.

Other poor typing habits which can lead to CRS include holding the left thumb extended out of the way and extending the fifth finger of either hand. These positions add more tension to the fingers and cause counter-muscular forces that must be overcome by the small muscles of the fingers, which are simultaneously alternating the rapid contractions and relaxations required by keyboard work.

PREVENTION

Above all, correct hand and finger position is essential. The ideal position is that of an old-school classical pianist (as opposed to some modern pianists who lean over the piano and rest their wrists on the edge of the piano keyboard). The following photo demonstrates how the fingers curve naturally and "drop" onto the keyboard rather than being forced down by muscle contraction. Proper technique may seem unnatural at first if the writer has been using poor technique, such as resting the hands on wrist rests, but the benefits will soon be evident.

Correct positioning of the keyboard so that it is slightly above the knees enhances the natural movement of the fingers and eases tension in the arms and shoulders. The keyboard that is posi-

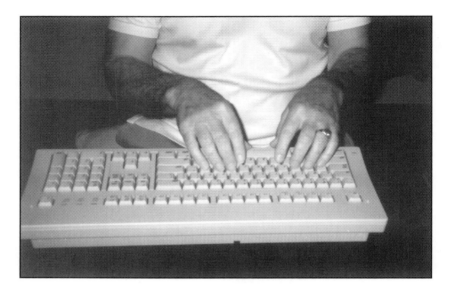

Relaxed, natural hand position without use of forearm rests or wrist rests. Slight outward cant of the hands. Neutral or slight downward droop of the wrists so the knuckles are slightly lower than the wrists. Elbow resting comfortably at the sides without holding the arm away from the body by the shoulder muscles. Wrist rest placed *under* the front of the keyboard to level the keyboard.

tioned flat instead of tilted up at the rear allows for better hand position. For those with small hands and short fingers, a smaller keyboard with less lateral spacing between keys lessens the degree of reach, but may contribute to other difficulties of the shoulders by reducing the movement of the arms.

To avoid CRS, relax the fingers and become aware of tension in the hands. Take measures to reduce muscle tightness in the fingers and hands. The following practice may be helpful: Instead of moving the fingers directly from one key to another, precede each keystroke with a brief period of complete relaxation. For instance, if the index finger of the right hand were to type "N U," the finger first types "N," relaxes, then types "U." Although it may seem awkward to the experienced typist, by slowing down and including periods of relaxation, speed and accuracy gradually improve, resulting in less tension in the muscles of the fingers and hands.

The thumb is vulnerable to several special problems. Forceful extension of the thumb to keep it out of the way places abnormal stress on the extensor tendon of the thumb, causing tendinitis (inflammation of the tendon). The writer experiences pain along the base of the thumb and wrist. The tendon may be tender to the touch and stretching the tendon may cause sharp pain. Treatment may be simple, such as avoiding abnormal postures of the thumb, or it may require more medical intervention, such as injection of anti-inflammatory drugs into the tendon sheath and occasionally immobilization with a splint or a cast. A condition called "trigger finger" of the thumb, a sticking or snapping of the thumb during ordinary movements, may cause the writer to think the thumb is awkward or paralyzed. This can also be treated with rest, immobilization, physical therapy, occasionally an injection of cortisone, or infrequently, surgery.

There are several easy ways to break bad habits and thereby reduce or avoid the need for any medical intervention. For example, if a writer is in the habit of holding the thumb in an extended position while typing, holding a ping pong ball, a quarter, or a similar object lightly in the web between the thumb and index finger will help the writer or computer worker change this undesirable posture. Similarly, holding a small ball of yarn, or something of similar size, in the curve of the little finger will pre-

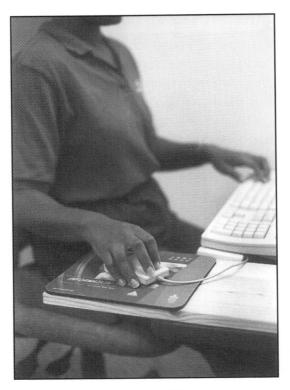

Mouse positioned to the side, making reaching unnecessary. Mouse is operated by rotating the arm at the shoulder rather than reaching.

vent its unconscious extension during keyboard use. Both exercises reduce counter-muscle tension in the hand and help it become as relaxed as possible. Watching oneself type using a mirror is probably the best way of correcting errors in technique.

When using the *mouse,* many computer workers hold the index finger straight and fully extended, pressing the mouse button with only the index finger pad, placing more strain on the fingers as well as the muscles of the hand and forearm. By using two fingers—usually the index and the middle finger together—on the mouse button, less effort is needed and muscle strain is reduced. Similarly, using two fingers on the "return," "delete," or any other large keys reduces the stress and fatigue of the fingers and forearm extensor muscles.

Squeezing the mouse while moving it also causes stress in the thumb and fingers, eventually resulting in tendinitis of the flexor tendons of the thumb. To avoid this, place the mouse where it is easily reached and operated without holding the arm extended at the shoulder and elbow. An extension attached to the desk or table that places the mouse at the side of the writer eliminates much of the static loading resulting from usual mouse placement. A six-inch board held to the surface of the table with clamps may suffice. (See photo on page 52.)

Use a mirror or video camera to check hand position and technique occasionally while writing. Many writers are surprised to find how often their hand position becomes awkward. A videotape can also demonstrate how poor posture adds tension and strain to the hand, especially the little fingers and the thumbs.

When starting to use the keyboard, warm up slowly. A few practice runs, the alphabet, or a few exercises done very slowly and easily prepare the fingers to work and to write. Develop a rhythm with a steady rate and controlled speed. Avoid sudden rushes of movement; keep even the most natural and easy combinations of keystrokes under control.

For those with persistent difficulty with the fingers, converting to an alternative arrangement of keys may be useful. The Dvorak or American Simplified Key arrangement places the most commonly used keys under the fingers in the middle row of keys, greatly reducing the motion of the fingers.* Those who convert to this system often find that fewer mistakes occur, which reduces the total number of keystrokes needed for a given task. Less finger motion and decreased force results in less swelling and soreness of the fingers, but it also reduces the movement of the arms and shoulders, increasing static loading of the upper arms. Many computer programs include the capability for custom or Dvorak key arrangements.

---

*A Dvorak keyboard is laid out as follows:

'	,	.	P	Y	F	G	C	R	L	/	=
A	O	E	U	I	D	H	T	N	S	-	
;	Q	J	K	X	B	M	W	V	Z		

7

The Hand

The hand has been a symbol of expressiveness since the beginning of time, and this continues with the hand used on the computer keyboard. In ancient Egyptian language, the term designating the hand was similar to that for the pillar, i.e., support or strength. In Islamic cultures, the hand is an amulet, a charm against evils. According to Berber thought, the hand signifies protection, authority, power, and strength, similar to the *manus* of the Romans, particularly the authority of the *pater familias* or of the emperor. In Jungian psychology, the hand is endowed with generative significance. The right hand is the rational, the conscious, the logical, and the virile; the left hand is the converse.

What is conceived in the mind is usually expressed by the hands:

"His mind and his hand went together, and what
he thought he uttered with that easiness that we
have scarce received from him a blot in his papers."
John Heminge and Henry Condell, preface to
First Folio of Shakespeare's Plays

Pain in the dorsum or top of the hand is a common form of discomfort in computer workers. Also,
many writers complain of tightness and swelling of
the hand, both the back of the hand and the palm.
The center of the palm, where the flexor tendons
traverse the length of the hand, may be tender due
to tendinitis or inflammation of the tendon sheaths
of the palm. Repetitive motion of a tendon in its
sheath in the palm leads to friction (not even the
body is perfect and friction or rubbing does occur),
microtrauma, and inflammation. Pain, tenderness,
and swelling may be felt in the palm under the
knuckle joints.

The proper position of the hand at the keyboard
is very similar to the position of hands resting in the
lap. When the keyboard is used properly, the position of the fingers does not change very much. Instead, the arms and shoulders move the hands forward, backward, and sideways to reach keys on near
and far rows. Very little reaching or lateral stretching of the fingers is either needed or desirable.

Pain and tenderness of the fleshy, muscular part of
palm at the base of the thumb and the muscular area
of the heel of the hand frequently occur and are probably due to persistent tension in the muscles caused
by holding the fingers apart in order to reach keys at
distances that cover the width of the keyboard, rather
than moving the hands freely from the shoulders.
Symptoms can be caused by neurovascular entrap-

ment anywhere along the course of the neurovascular structures (i.e., nerve and blood vessels) of the neck or upper extremity, although discomfort may be felt only in the hands.

On examination of the hands findings other than tenderness of the muscle areas of the hand and pain during motion are often meager. Swelling is all but immeasurable by any ordinary clinical means. Weakness of grip can occur when the tissues of the hands are inflamed and painful. In some instances a doctor may discover the existence of tendon cysts, which are fluid-filled sacs found along the course of a tendon, especially at the top of the wrist and the base of the thumb. These are the result of repetitive motions of the fingers and occur on the dorsum of the hand or in the palm, especially under the knuckle joints.

CAUSE

Repetitive, rapid movements can cause increased friction of the tendons in their sheaths, leading to swelling and increased pressure due to confinement of muscles, tendons, and nerves in the tight spaces and compartments of the hand. The hand was "designed" to grasp and to allow man to manipulate large objects and swing from trees, but not to handle paper or to make rapid, repeated movements on the keyboard. Static loading of the small muscles of the hand occurs when the fingers are held wide apart and results in additional tension, fatigue, and pain.

PREVENTION

Prevention focuses on relaxed movements of the hands and fingers, which is easier to say than to do. The relaxation techniques noted in chapter 14 can also be helpful for the hand. Instead of holding the fingers wide apart ready to reach for keys at the extremes of the keyboard, relax the hands so the fingers fall together as if the hand were resting in the writer's lap. Reach with motions of the shoulders and arms, not the fingers. This is a difficult habit to break, but the benefits are certainly worth it.

The correct position of the hands and fingers is of paramount importance. With a gentle curve of the fingers and relaxed movement of the arms, writers can avoid lateral stretching of the fingers. For those who have unusually short fifth fingers (making reaching keys while the wrist is frozen to a wrist rest even more difficult), a smaller keyboard may help, but smaller keyboards are not generally available and have their own inherent risks. A better solution is to move the hand about the keyboard by initiating movement from the shoulders rather than stretching with the fingers.

The Dvorak key arrangement was developed to reduce the movement of the fingers and the frequency of stretches of the intrinsic muscles of the hand while typing. The Dvorak key arrangement is gaining acceptance, and those who have adopted it find it much easier on the fingers and hands than the conventional QWERTY keyboard. Users also report that conversion to the Dvorak key arrangement is learned with surprisingly little difficulty.

Be good to your hands. Do not start to write if the hands and fingers feel cold or clammy. Warm and gently stretch the hands and forearms. When away from writing, be careful that the hands don't fall prey to other misfortunes. The hands are as muscular as the biceps, thighs, or back; they too need their time for rest.

TREATMENT

- Warm the hands and forearms before starting to write and as needed during computer use to increase blood flow and reduce muscle tightness.

- Gently massage the muscles of the base of the thumb and heel of the hand.

- Cool down after a period of writing. Use ice packs or cold water on the hands like a baseball pitcher or a handball player after a game.

- When resting during or after a period of writing, allow the hands to rest in the lap or on the table turned partially toward a palms-up position so that they are not fully turned down flat (pronated) in the same position as at the keyboard. A change in posture of the forearms relaxes and lessens static tension of the hands and forearms.

8

The Wrist

The firm, iron wrist of the soldier or wrestler can be compared to the limber wrist of the dancer or artist to provide ample illustration of the expressive distinctiveness of the wrist. The computer keyboard adds both expressive ability and attendant risks.

Problems and complaints about the wrists account for as much as 20 percent of worker's compensation claims. Complaints of pain, stiffness, and swelling of the top (dorsum) and the underside (volar) of the wrist occur frequently in the computer worker. The wrist is especially vulnerable to developing symptoms in computer workers because the long tendons of the muscles of the forearm traverse both the top and underside of the wrist all the way to the fingers. The tendons and related structures are richly endowed with pain fibers, so what might appear to be a small injury tends to cause intense pain.

Limited flexion or extension of the wrist is the

most common abnormality and usually reflects tightness of the muscles of the forearm. Tendinitis of the wrist causes tenderness along the course of the tendon, pain and restricted movement of the tendon, and pain with passive stretching of the tendon. Inflammation of tendons may occur at the muscle and tendon junction, along the course of the tendon itself, or where the tendon attaches to bone. Tenderness over the dorsum and underside of the wrist are present when the tendons and related structures (such as the tendon sheaths, which allow smooth motions of tendons) are inflamed.

Tenderness may occur at other prominent points, such as over the bones at the heel of the hand near the thumb side of the wrist or the bony prominence at the little-finger side of the wrist. These, too, are due to excessive pressure or repeated stress and static loading while holding the wrists and hands firmly in one position over long periods of time, often in postures that put excessive strain on these small structures.

Although symptoms are more common at the dorsum, other areas of the wrist may also be tender. Tenderness of the volar side of the wrist may extend toward the muscles of the forearm which flex the fingers. Extension of the wrist (bending it back toward the upper side of the forearm) may be restricted and cause pulling and pain in the forearm muscles. Occasionally, if the tendons are extremely irritated and inflamed, swelling occurs and a rough or "scratchy" sensation can be felt by the patient and observed by the examiner when the fingers are flexed.

Tendon cysts may develop on either side of the wrist in response to over-use, but these cysts are generally not harmful nor do they limit the use of the hands. We recommend a physician examine any unusual swelling of the wrist or hand noted by the computer worker.

CAUSE

The cause of pain in the wrists is nearly always overuse. Rapid, repetitive use of the fingers causes friction of the tendons and tendon sheath. Repetitive motion combined with abnormal posture of the wrists (such as the wrists flexed upward) and further aggravated by twisting the wrist (ulnar deviation), causes lateral pressure on the tissues that retain tendons in their normal positions, resulting in a high degree of friction and microtrauma to the tendons and their delicate surrounding tissues. Such abnormal lateral strain is further provoked by internal rotation of the wrists, that is, rotating the wrists to a position with the palms down (pronation), a common keyboard posture.

A special hazard of the wrists occurs when the writer, clerk, supervisor, or trouble-shooter leans on his or her wrists on the wrist rest while standing and using the keyboard, causing an extraordinary forced extension of the wrists. This posture puts inordinate strain on the flexor tendons on the underside of the wrists as well as an abnormal angle of forces on the extensor tendons on top of the wrists. It may also compress the nerves and blood vessels which traverse the wrist.

The use of a mouse may also cause difficulty with the wrist. If the mouse is placed on a mouse pad that is lower than the keyboard, the wrist may be held extended, or bent upward. If the mouse is too high, the shoulder is elevated, increasing tightness in the neck muscles and overextending the wrist. While using the mouse, the writer must wait for the computer to process data, during which time, the wrist remains in an undesirable, extended position with the fingers held out straight.

PREVENTION

Prevention of wrist problems is extremely important, because once symptoms of pain and tightness develop, a great deal of inflammation of the fine structures of the wrist has already occurred. Continued use of the wrists and hands when they are inflamed risks further tissue injury.

Of primary importance is proper wrist posture, which, unfortunately, is seldom seen even in the most experienced writer or computer worker. The simplicity of the keyboard gives the illusion that most any wrist or hand position can be maintained without penalty, but the only desirable and safe position of the hand is with the wrists held high, "floating" above the keyboard. The best posture of the wrist and hand positions the fingers, tendons of the back of the hand, and the forearm in a nearly straight line as seen from the side, avoiding undesirable sharp angles of the tendons at the wrist. The wrist should be held in a neutral position with neither flexion nor extension. A slight downward droop of the wrists of no more than 10 to 15 degrees can lessen sideways pressure on the soft tissues of the wrist and is acceptable. A slight outward cant or rotation of the wrists so that the little-finger side of the hand is a little closer to the keyboard than the

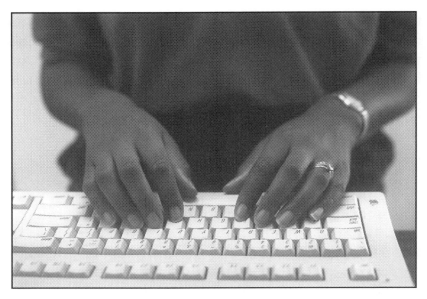

Wrist and hand position relaxed with no hazardous angles. Wrists slightly canted outward to relax the forearms.

thumb side also reduces strain in the wrist and forearm. The best and safest position of the wrist (as shown in the photograph above) also relaxes the muscles of the forearms.

Avoid holding the wrists and hands still in one position for long periods. Do not use wrist rests or other pads that restrict the floating motion of the hands over the keyboard. The computer worker may unconsciously lean on the wrist rests, producing pressure on the structures of the wrist, contributing to further abnormal postures, making the writer subject his hands and wrists to greater hazard. If the writer chooses to write standing up, like Hemingway, raise the keyboard to a proper and reasonable height to avoid abnormal and harmful postures of the wrists and hands.

Do not allow a computer mouse to remain lower

than the keyboard. Raise the mouse on a book or a package of paper to a height that allows the wrist to remain in a neutral position. This will reduce friction on the wrist tendons. Avoid squeezing the mouse excessively; only a light touch is needed to move it. While the computer responds to the commands from the mouse, drop the hands into the lap and allow them to rest a few moments.

TREATMENT

Rest is the cornerstone of the treatment of tendinitis. The first and most important step toward cure is suspension of activity. This is followed by stretching the muscles and tendons, and finally, gradually strengthening the muscle.

- Change the position of the wrists and hands.

- Gently massage the wrists and hands.

- Gently flex and extend the wrist during rest breaks.

- Keep the elbows relaxed and close to the sides. Wrist position and elbow position are intimately related.

- Again, *avoid* the use of wrist rests while writing! Leaning on the wrists while they are on the wrist rest can become a habit, especially with fatigue or stress. Let the hands float over the keyboard. Do not anchor them in one place for long periods. When the wrists are anchored in place, additional strain is placed on fingers that must reach for out-of-the-way keys, contributing to static loading of the muscles of the arms and shoulders. With a little practice, the writer can learn to reach these keys readily by moving the arms rather than by reaching with the fingers.

To break the habit of using a wrist rest, the writer can practice moving over the keyboard without typing so the arms and shoulders are freed from their fixed position, then adopt these motions when using the keyboard.

Formerly, secretaries sat forward on their chairs, back straight, arms to their sides, typing on mechanical typewriters in what is still the safest posture for writers. They moved. They typed with the tips of the fingers and frequently changed positions—using the return lever and placing a new piece of paper in the typewriter carriage. They took breaks at the water cooler. They did not suffer from the epidemic of upper-extremity troubles that afflict modern computer keyboard workers, who become caught up in the task of creation, intent on their work, often forgetting safe positions of the wrist or hand, and falling into harmful, habitual postures. The computer can outlast the most durable keyboarder. The writer, if not on guard, can stay at the computer until forced to stop from exhaustion or unbearable pain.

Take care of your hands and wrists when away from the computer keyboard. Do not lean on the hands with the wrists sharply flexed or extended at any time.

Many people clench their fists at night, or hold their wrists sharply flexed or extended while asleep, applying pressure-stress on the wrists and causing discomfort. A towel may be wrapped around the wrists or a soft material may be fashioned to keep the wrists and hands from harmful, end-range motion of the joints during the night. Wrist splints may be needed temporarily to maintain a neutral position of the wrists while asleep.

Do not use the hands and wrists as hammers, or as a pry, or for twisting and wringing movements. Avoid hard wrenching wrist movements in any direction. Hands and wrists are as important to the writer as the vocal cords are to an opera singer, the elbow to a baseball pitcher, or the hamstring to a sprinter. It may be imagination and creativity that make a writer, but it is the hands and arms that do the writing.

CARPAL TUNNEL SYNDROME

One of the most widely known risks of writing and using the computer keyboard is carpal tunnel syndrome, one of the "nerve entrapment" conditions that affects the upper extremity. Those who perform repetitive motions of the hand and wrists, such as meat packers, writers, grocery checkers, and keyboard workers, are especially prone to this disorder, which is caused by pressure on the median nerve at the underside of the wrist.

Anatomy

The carpal tunnel is about one centimeter in diameter and bounded on three sides by the bones of the wrist, which form an arch. Passing through the arch are nine tendons that flex the fingers and a branch of the median nerve that supplies sensation to the thumb, index, middle, and the inside of the ring fingers. The carpal ligament encloses the tunnel on the underside of the wrist. Thus, the carpal tunnel is bound on all sides by bony or ligamentous structures that are firm and do not expand when swelling occurs inside the canal. Activities and postures of the wrist that increase pressure within the canal exert an abnormal force on the tissues located there. Of these tissues, the median nerve is the most pressure sensitive. An increase in pressure, then, causes symptoms such as numbness, tingling, and loss of sensation of the thumb, index, middle, and ring fingers. If the pressure on the median nerve continues, the thumb's ability to pinch with the index finger is weakened.

Complaints include numbness, tingling, burning, or a buzzing-electric feeling in the hand, as well as a decreased or absent sensation of the fingers. These result from pressure and irritation of the median nerve in the carpal tunnel. Only one or two fingers may feel numb or have loss of sensation, but if damage is severe and prolonged, all four fingers supplied with nerve function by the median nerve may become affected. Symptoms tend to occur during activities that are associated with either sustained flexion or extension of the wrist, such as driving, holding a book or newspaper, and repetitive use of the hands while typing, cutting with scissors, and sleeping. Carpal tunnel syndrome may accompany any condition that causes increased "crowding" or pressure in the carpal tunnel, such as a previous fracture of the wrist, pregnancy, hypothyroidism, rheumatoid arthritis, and a few other, less common conditions.

On examination, the findings in carpal tunnel syndrome include decreased sensation of the palmar side of the fingers of the thumb, index finger, middle finger, and the inside of the ring finger and decreased pinch strength between the thumb and index fingers. In extreme cases, loss of muscle bulk of the thumb side of the hand occurs. Symptoms of numbness and tingling are reproduced by holding the wrist in full flexion or full extension for two minutes. Tapping lightly on the palmar surface of the wrist over the course of the median nerve may cause tingling or electric sensation into the fingers due to irritability of the median nerve in the carpal tunnel. Special tests, such as the electromyogram (EMG), may show a delay in conduction of the nerve impulse across the carpal ligament of the wrist.

Cause

Carpal tunnel syndrome is caused by pressure at the wrist on the median nerve. Pressure within the carpal tunnel is greatly increased by repetitive movement of the tendons located there, and pressure is further increased if the wrists are extended or bent toward the top of the hand, and also by ulnar deviation of the wrists (turning the hand toward the little-finger side).

Musculotendon symptoms of the forearm and hand (such as restriction of finger and wrist motion due to shortening of the muscles, as well as complaints of tightness or weakness) are much more common than nerve compression symptoms (numbness and tingling) in the carpal tunnel. Carpal tunnel syndrome appears to be preceded by musculotendon problems, which eventually lead to the nerve compression disorder. Carpal tunnel-like symptoms may also be caused by compression of nerves and/or blood vessels in the neck, shoulder, and upper chest cage. These disorders may be a more frequent cause of nerve compression symptoms in the hand of the writer than of carpal tunnel syndrome itself.

Entrapment of the median nerve in the forearm near the elbow may give symptoms and findings identical to carpal tunnel syndrome. In this case, the median nerve is entrapped by the pronator muscle, which turns the hand toward a palm-down position.

Prevention

Carpal tunnel syndrome can be avoided in most instances. Since the musculotendinous component of repetitive strain injury is many times more frequent than the nerve component, proper positioning of the fingers, wrists, and forearms is of foremost importance in prevention. To reduce pressure in the carpal tunnel:

- Avoid unnecessary repetitions of an activity or action.

- Avoid overly hard gripping with the hands.

- Avoid sharply flexed and extended positions of the wrists.

- Avoid deviation of the wrist toward the heel of the hand.

- Avoid clenching the hands. Use a relaxed wrist position while driving or holding a book or newspaper, and especially at night, to avoid prolonged contraction of the forearm muscles.

- Avoid tucking the hand into the neck or against the chest with the wrist sharply bent in flexion or extension during sleep. Some writers need to wrap their hand in towel splints or have hand splints custom-made to keep the wrists and hands in proper position during the night.

- Avoid leaning on the hands with pressure on the palms. Be aware and use correct wrist positioning.

Once carpal tunnel syndrome has been diagnosed, a course of physical and/or occupational therapy may be in order, and improvement can occur within just four weeks. If these measures do not suffice to relieve the symptoms, surgery to sever the carpal ligament may be required. Injections of a small amount of a cortisone-like medicine into the carpal tunnel to decrease swelling are often beneficial and may give temporary or long-lasting relief.

Carpal tunnel syndrome may be intermittent and does not always require injection or surgery. Provided symptoms are not too severe, if enough time for rest and relief from abuse is granted the swelling within the carpal tunnel may recede of its own accord.

Give your carpal tunnel a chance: When writing hold the wrists in a neutral or near neutral position, and avoid extension and ulnar deviation of the wrists.

OTHER NERVE ENTRAPMENT SYNDROMES

The ulnar nerve may become compressed at the elbow, causing complaints of numbness of the ring and little fingers. The symptoms of nerve entrapment include numbness, tingling, and weakness. Pain is not a prominent complaint. Stretching of the ulnar nerve at the elbow may be responsible for pressure on the ulnar nerve, which may be caused or aggravated by prolonged flexion of the elbow while at work. Limit elbow flexion to no more than ninety degrees and preferably somewhat greater so that the wrist is slightly lower than the elbow while at the computer. Stretching the ulnar nerve may be aggravated by holding the elbows flexed tightly at night. In this case, a towel splint about the elbow and arm may be necessary for maintaining a comfortable posture of the elbow at night.

The other major nerve of the forearm and hand is the radial nerve. It is seldom involved in entrapments, but when entrapped, it causes numbness and tingling over the upper part of the wrist and hand. Entrapment may occur higher in the arm at the shoulder or as the nerves lie over the ribs in the "thoracic outlet" or as they branch near the cervical spine. The symptoms of thoracic outlet syndrome are highly variable and tend to be intermittent. They are markedly accentuated by abnormal postures at the keyboard, such as the head jutting forward and the shoulders up and rounded forward. Diagnosis relies on physical findings, since there is no reliable test for this condition.

Another common ailment involves weakness of the scapular muscles of the shoulder due to nerve compression at the thoracic outlet (where the nerves of the neck and blood vessels from the chest pass through the upper part of the chest). Treatment with physical therapy is usually successful, but requires sessions two to three times per week for six to eight weeks or longer. Those with thoracic outlet syndrome have muscle tightness of the neck and drooping, rounded shoulders. These are problems that often require specialized care, and will not be covered here.

"Adverse neural tissue tension" is a recently recognized disorder that is thought to be due to nerve tension or lack of tissue pliability about the nerve at any point along its path. Symptoms are often similar to those of other nerve entrapment problems of the upper extremity—pain, stiffness, numbness, and muscular tightness—but do not always occur in the usual anatomical patterns and may present even fewer physical findings than do other problems of the upper extremity. The diagnosis can be established by certain maneuvers that stretch the nerve along its course.

Normally, the nerve lies within and moves lengthwise along with the artery and vein in the neurovascular bundle, but when adverse neural tissue tension is present (often due to repetitive use or trauma), the nerve is thought to be "bound down" and irritable. A poor sitting position at the computer such as with the head forward and the shoulders rounded is especially liable to place pressure on the nerves at the shoulder and thoracic outlet, contributing to neural tension.

Treatment must be carried out under the supervision of an experienced physical therapist who is trained in this particular discipline.

9

The Forearm

"The forearm . . . consists of two bones lying along-
side each other, but touching only at the ends."
William Paley, *Natural Theology*

Modern computer workers may at times wish they had
forearms the size of Popeye's, because much of the effort of writing and use of the computer keyboard is felt
there. It takes something other than a can of spinach
and a powerful grip, however, to manage the keyboard.

The forearm is one of the most troublesome
areas for the writer. Discomfort and pain in the
forearms tend to be diffuse and not localized to particular spots or discrete locations. Early symptoms
usually include muscle tightness, pain, and soreness rather than numbness or tingling. Weakness of
the forearm muscles is experienced as weakness in
the hands and wrists; the writer drops objects, or
cannot open jars, car doors, and the like.

Although muscle tightness and stiffness occur in the muscle groups of the underside of the forearm (the muscles that flex the wrist and the long muscles that flex the fingers), pain tends to be located more toward the wrist at the musculotendinous junction. A sensation of fullness or swelling along with wrist extension restrictions occur. Complaints of problems related to the volar aspect (the underside) of the forearm are less common than those of the extensor (top or outside) forearm. The extensor muscles, however, are often the site of aching pain, muscular soreness, tightness, and stiffness severe enough to cause the writer to seek medical advice. It is the pain in this area that often restricts the amount of writing that can be tolerated. When injured and inflamed these muscles become tight and shortened, preventing the normal full, painless flexion of the wrist and fingers. Grasping, carrying, and twisting motions of the wrist and forearm, and flexion or extension of the fingers and/or wrist cause much of the discomfort. The arms may feel weak and heavy, and the writer may lack endurance due to pain and/or weakness. Sustained use of the hands may increase pain and weakness to the point that the writer is forced to stop using the keyboard entirely for a time.

FINDINGS ON EXAMINATION

The muscles of the forearm, especially the extensor muscles, may be tender and sore to touch or massage, and feel firm and not relaxed. Pinching or rolling the skin-fold over the forearm muscles may cause intense, burning pain, which may also be brought out by the examiner holding the wrist firm while the writer tries to forcefully extend, flex, or twist it against resistance. Passive flexion of the wrist may be restricted because of shortening of the musculotendinous unit of the forearm muscles. The forearm may feel swollen, but appear normal on examination.

CAUSE

Causes of pain and discomfort of the forearm include a combination of rapid, repetitive movements and static loading. In order to stabilize the wrist while at the keyboard, the forearm muscles must remain contracted and stationary for long periods of time. Other muscles of the forearm must contract and relax, or relax against resistance, in rapid, alternating motions thousands of times during a day. Blood flow to the forearm muscles increases with use, which over time results in swelling. The swelling causes back-pressure on blood flow, interfering with adequate oxygen supply to the muscles and soft tissues. They become "ischemic"; blood supply is reduced and metabolic waste removal is impaired. The end result is scarring and shortening of the muscles and tendons of the forearm. The shortened, ischemic muscles and tendons must overcome greater and greater resistance with more and more injury to the small muscle fibers, resulting in more scarring: a vicious and destructive cycle.

PREVENTION

Avoiding injury begins with an awareness of the risks of improper positioning, posture, and technique. Proper posture of the wrists and fingers is a fundamental principle in the health of the forearms, because abnormal posture of the wrists combined with rapid movements of the tendons increase the work of the already compromised forearm muscles.

Begin slowly with a *warm-up* before starting a period of writing, just like an athlete. Gently *stretch* the muscles and tendons of the forearm, wrist, and hands. *Massage* the muscles of the forearm and hand. The forearms are to the writer as the hamstring muscles are to a sprinter. Although it may seem elementary to experienced writers and keyboard workers, doing a few basic exercises or the alphabet in a slow, controlled manner before actually writing helps to attain good posture and establish a comfortable, relaxed rhythm.

Once the day's writing has begun, be certain to take breaks away from your workstation of at least a few minutes in length. Although the computer will never stop because you are typing too fast, software is available that will allow you to program it to shut off for a rest period every hour or so. During this rest period learn to relax the muscles of the forearm, let the wrists droop. Next, hold arms over head and gently wiggle the fingers to help reduce swelling.

At night, make sure the hands are not clenched tightly so that the muscles of the hands and forearms are fatigued and stressed in the morning. Ensuring that the hands are not clenched before falling asleep is usually sufficient to prevent clenching during the night. A towel splint or other such device can be used for this purpose.

Proper positioning of the wrists during writing with the hands slightly drooped and the wrists canted or rotated slightly outward (so that the little finger is slightly closer to the keyboard) lessens the static tension of the wrist, stabilizing muscles of the forearm and reducing the overall work of the forearm muscles. This in turn reduces the demand on blood supply, lessening swelling and ischemia. Muscle relaxation of the forearms can be accomplished by gently flopping the wrist back and forth.

Optimum sitting posture is essential to preventing injury. The forearms and arms are held with the arms relaxed against the sides and the forearms parallel to the floor. The wrists are held about the same height as the elbows or slightly lower. Proper alignment of the spine, shoulders, hands, and wrists, along with proper breathing patterns, can reduce tension in the forearms to a minimum. Any posture that is maintained for long periods eventually becomes uncomfortable and painful, and change of position becomes essential even if the posture is optimal. Therefore, the writer must be on guard against poor postures because even the most harmful ones may feel comfortable for a short time, but if maintained, they add to the cumulative injury.

Avoid carrying heavy briefcases or other heavy objects long distances, as this forces the forearm muscles into sustained contraction, adding to their tension, fatigue, and strain.

Prevention of prolonged or excessive muscle tension and poor postures of the trunk, arms, and forearms is difficult because the writer focuses on what he or she is writing by excluding both external distractions and internal stimuli. The writer's wrists and hands may assume awkward, harmful positions without the writer being aware of it.

TREATMENT

Treatment begins with an awareness of the risks writers take by continuing to write after the first discomforts appear. All too often, we tend to deny that there is anything wrong. Pay attention to early warnings such as heaviness of the arms, tightness or swelling of the forearms, soreness about the wrists. If the soreness persists after a short period of rest, do not wait for more troublesome symptoms to arise. Seek help.

By far the most important aspect of treatment is *rest* of the hands and arms. Not only rest from writing, but rest from other sustained use, repetitive motions, gripping, twisting, etc. Rest allows the swelling of small, soft tissues to subside with increased circulation and blood supply. Rest from writing or the computer keyboard permits healing of microtrauma to the tendons and related tissues. Rest may need to be prolonged, that is, weeks and possibly months or longer in some instances.

Gentle, careful *stretching* under the supervision of a therapist skilled in the treatment of these problems is essential. Improper, overly vigorous stretching exercise harms the muscle and becomes detrimental to recovery. Adding stretching to a daily routine will be beneficial throughout the professional lifetime of the writer. The writer is cautioned to stretch gently and regularly, even when symptoms of over-use are not being experienced. Stretch both the flexor and the extensor muscles of the forearm, and stretch in a manner that does not cause pain at the time or undue stiffness and pain afterward.

A gentle *massage* of the extensor muscles of the forearm can be performed with the heel of the other hand. Deep massage of the muscles stretches the muscle and must be performed by a skilled physical therapist. *Skin-fold massage* of the loose skin over tight, tender forearm muscles lessens soreness. This type of massage is performed by lifting the loose fold of skin between the base of the thumb and the fingers and rolling it gently. Initially, the skin may seem extremely tender and there may be a burning sensation, but this discomfort will pass and relief should be obtained.

If the forearms feel swollen or tight, using ice or letting cold water run over them as often as necessary may greatly lessen discomfort, pain, and stiffness. Ice is used no more than one minute at a time and no more often than every thirty minutes. Cold packs can be applied for ten to twenty minutes at a time as often as every two hours. Some individuals are advised not use ice if they have circulation or other cold-sensitive illnesses.

Contrast baths help to relieve pain and reduce swelling of the soft tissues of the forearm. These are performed by alternate use of warm and cold water: The warm water should range from 100 to 102 degrees Fahrenheit, and the cold water should be about 40 degrees Fahrenheit (cold tap water). A double sink, with one side cold and the other side hot, is convenient for contrast baths of the hands. Care must be taken that the warm water is not too hot and does not cool off during the procedure. Immerse the hands at least halfway from the wrist to the elbow.

Place the hands in the warm bath first for a period of five minutes, and then one minute in the cold water. Then three minutes in the warm, followed by one minute in the cold. Repeat for a total of fifteen to twenty minutes. Contrast baths can be done several times a day if needed.

An alternate method is to warm the hands in warm water until comfortably warm, then immerse the hand in cold water until uncomfortably cold, and repeat several cycles, ending in the warm water. This abbreviated method is useful when the writer or computer worker is at work, as it can be performed during breaks, during the lunch break, and after the work day.

A series of contrast baths should begin and end in warm water. At times, however, immersing the hands in cold water alone is sufficient, especially if the hands feel puffy or swollen.

If the writer or computer worker has any condition that is heat or cold sensitive, do not perform contrast baths or apply heat or cold to the hands unless approved by a physician.

Mild analgesic medicines (such as aspirin, acetaminophen, ibuprofen, etc.) may be helpful if the pain and soreness is especially uncomfortable, but these medicines are to be used only to lessen resting pain and discomfort, and *not* to allow the writer to "keep going."

Splints used during rest periods relax the muscles of the forearm when away from the keyboard. Generally, splints are limited to short-term use in acute injury to lessen pain and inflammation and are not recommended for prolonged use. The muscle and tendon tissues respond better to gradual, gentle stretching followed by slow, progressive strengthening.

10

The Elbow

"One rub'd his elboe thus, and fleer'd and swore."
William Shakespeare, *Love's Labor Lost*

Several distinct sites near the elbow can be troublesome for the computer worker. Pain and tenderness
are the principal complaint related to the elbow.
The soft tissue at the inside of the elbow and bony
structures at the outside, where the overlying skin
does not provide very much padding, are especially
vulnerable to mild trauma in everyday activities.
When coupled with the stress of musculotendinous
attachments at these same sites, elbow pain and
soreness may become intense. The pain may not be
localized, because it is sometimes due to inflammation in the area of the proximal radio-ulnar joint,
which lies under the muscles of the forearm close to
the elbow. Pain may be present much of the time
and usually worsens with use. When severe, pain in

the elbow may interfere with the writer's ability to write and grasp, and may disturb the writer's sleep.

Pain and inflammation—what is often called "tennis elbow"—frequently occurs at the lateral epicondyle, the bony point at the outside of the elbow. This is one of the sites where the muscles and tendons of the forearm attach to the humerus, the bone which forms the upper arm and therefore ends at the elbow. This area is vulnerable to trauma and is a common site of pain and tenderness; it is always the spot that gets bumped. Use of the hands, especially repetitive grasping and movements in which the wrists and fingers are extended, aggravates pain in the elbow as the epicondyle becomes inflamed. Since this bony prominence has little soft tissue overlying it, it is easy to palpate and may be quite tender.

The medial epicondyle, the bony prominence at the inside aspect of the elbow, is less likely to cause difficulty for the writer, but it occasionally can be painful as a result of the stress of grasping and repetitive activities that flex the wrist and fingers. It is not unusual for both the lateral and medial epicondyle to be tender and painful at the same time.

The proximal radio-humeral joint, the joint where the radius bone of the forearm rotates in its socket near the elbow, is located under the muscular, fleshy part of the upper side (extensor) of the forearm near the junction with the elbow. The only movement of this joint occurs when the forearm and wrist twist or rotate so the palm faces either up or down. When this joint is inflamed, it causes a deep ache in the upper forearm or elbow. Deep palpation over the radial head (the end of the radius bone of the forearm nearest the elbow) usually elicits marked tenderness.

Grasping and twisting with the wrist and hand can cause or aggravate inflammation of this joint.

FINDINGS ON EXAMINATION

Findings of slight swelling over the bony prominences of the elbow may be present, but often there is only tenderness. Tenderness may be quite marked, causing the writer to wince when the epicondyle is bumped or to protect the area when it is palpated during examination. Those individuals with an increased "carrying angle" (the angle formed by the upper arm and the forearm at the elbow when the arm is allowed to hang from the shoulder—not everyone's arm makes a straight line) are especially subject to abnormal postures of the arms and wrists when at the keyboard. Often the elbows are held away from the sides of the chest, causing static loading of the shoulder muscles. Those with an increased carrying angle of the elbow often have hyperextensibility of the fingers (overly limber joints).

The cause of distress at the various sites of the elbow tend to be similar: repetitive stress on the tendinous attachments of the forearm muscles to the bone, especially due to activities involving grasping, twisting, and carrying, or any activity associated with prolonged gripping.

PREVENTION

Prevention of difficulties at the elbow requires avoiding sudden, hard use of the hands and forearms in squeezing, pruning, clipping, lifting, pushing and pulling movements, or using a pair of pliers or screwdriver, especially when the writer is not accustomed to these activities. The use of appropriate tools and devices to reduce excessive torqueing (twisting) and static loading of these musculotendinous structures also reduces mechanical stress. Allowing the wrists and forearms to rotate outward somewhat while using the keyboard reduces the internal resting tension of the forearm muscles that stabilize the wrist.

A negative-tilt keyboard, that is, one with the edge of keyboard away from the writer lower than the edge closest to the writer, opens the angle of the elbow somewhat and reduces the risk of nerve injury at the elbow. It also lessens the tension of the arm muscles and frees the use of the shoulders.

TREATMENT

Treatment for inflammation of the epicondyle (epicondylitis of the elbow) may either be very simple or it may take some doing. Often application of heat to the affected area gives relief from soreness and tenderness. However, heat must be moderate so as not to injure the skin. To prevent heat injury, heat should not be applied more than ten or fifteen minutes at a time (longer periods of application may increase swelling and aggravate pain).

For localized pain and tenderness, ice applied to the area may relieve pain better than heat or other measures. As with heat, ice should not be held to the area more than a few minutes at a time. Convenient methods for local application of ice include ice cubes in a plastic bag separated from the skin by a damp cloth or a paper cup filled with water that has been allowed to freeze.

Time and rest of the forearm muscles may be the best treatment. Occasionally, physical therapy is necessary to properly retrain the muscles and to improve muscle tone and flexibility. Infrequently, injection of a local anesthetic alone or with a small amount of cortisone may be required to obtain relief of pain of epicondylitis of the elbow.

11

The Shoulder

"He whipped his horses . . . and put his shoulder
to the wheel."
Robert Burton, *Democritus to the Reader*

The shoulder joint is extremely complicated and
will be dealt with here only as it affects writers and
the use of the computer keyboard. Motions of the
shoulder are complex, and pain from the shoulder
joint and associated structures may be felt in areas
somewhat distant from the shoulder itself. On the
other hand, causes of pain arising some distance
from the chest and even within the abdomen may
refer pain to the shoulder.

Complaints of pain in the shoulder are difficult to
localize. Discomfort is often felt over a large area
and can be almost impossible to pin down to a specific location. Writers seeking medical advice seldom
complain about the shoulder itself, but many sites of

tenderness in that area are often found on physical examination. This occurs even though the principle area of pain may be elsewhere in the upper extremity. The most common complaints of discomfort are stiffness, aching, limited motion, and fatigue of the arms and shoulder muscles.

FINDINGS ON EXAMINATION

Findings on examination may include tenderness over several tendon areas, especially over the top of the shoulder, behind the shoulder, and the front of the shoulder. Bursitis, an inflammation of a bursa or small pouch of tissue that facilitates motion of the shoulder (and most joints), causes pain to be felt at the side of the shoulder and to the outer side of the shoulder and upper arm. Pain and tenderness are often accompanied by tightness or limited motions of the shoulder muscles and shortening of the pectoral muscles of the upper front of the chest. This shortening usually does not cause symptoms directly, but tenderness is present on examination in many cases. Tight pectoral muscles lead to abnormal postures of the shoulders and neck.

Tender points along the side of the shoulder blade (scapula) or at the "superior scapular angle" located between the shoulder blade and the base of the neck are also common findings. Tender points in the trapezius muscle over the top of the shoulder, along with tenderness of the loose fold of skin over the muscles about the shoulder, the upper trapezius muscle area, and the base of the neck frequently accompany pain and tenderness of other areas of the upper extremity.

CAUSE

The principal cause of pain in the shoulders of writers and computer workers is poor posture and static loading of the shoulder muscles due to a lack of movement. Increased tension and static loading of the muscles of the shoulders causes shortness and tightness of the front, upper chest and shoulder blade muscles. Even a slight forward angle or forward flexion of the shoulders greatly increases tension and fatigue of the shoulder muscles. In addition, improper breathing by over-using the ribs and chest cage, instead of abdominal/diaphragmatic breathing, also causes tightness of the muscles of the neck.

The *mouse-shoulder syndrome* is an insidious problem of the writer who uses the mouse a great deal, such as using the spell-checker on a long document. If the mouse is to the side of the keyboard, as it nearly always is, holding the arm unsupported to the side for long periods causes muscle fatigue pain of the entire shoulder through prolonged static loading. Prolonged extension of either shoulder produces static loading of both shoulders since the opposite spinal posture muscles counterbalance the weight of the arm being held outstretched. Extensive use of the mouse may cause finger extensor tendinitis, carpal tunnel syndrome, and neck and shoulder muscle pain.

PREVENTION

- Move. Sway rhythmically like a musician. Raise your arms after entering an emphatic period or exclamation point, like a pianist accenting a note.

- Posture! Posture! Posture! The chair and its arrangement, the height of the keyboard, and the location of the monitor all contribute to static loading of the postural muscles of the back, neck, and shoulders. Those with poor posture at the keyboard usually also exhibit poor posture during other activities. Posture, however, is more important to the health of the computer worker than most other considerations.

- Rotate the shoulders forward, up, back, and down—in the final position, you should look like a soldier standing rigidly at attention. When the shoulders slump forward and up, the pectoral muscles shorten, and abnormal tension is placed on the nerves of the neck and shoulders, causing static loading of the muscles of the neck.

Do *not* use a wrist rest or a forearm rest. Instead, allow the arms to move freely over the entire keyboard. Because workers tend to lean on them, wrist rests contribute to the tendency to a slumped sitting posture with the shoulders forward and elevated, and the head craned forward. They also limit arm motion, causing static loading, and they place the wrists in an extended position, instead of the desired neutral one. Move the arms at the shoulders to reach for keys, and do not reach with the fingers while the wrists are frozen in place. Having the wrists elevated, *not* on a wrist rest, aids both the fingers and the shoulders. Use wrist rests or forearm rests only while taking a break from using the keyboard, if at all. They have no function during the time the computer worker is actually using the keyboard.

Take regular, spaced breaks and rests even if for only a few minutes, and perform range-of-motion movements of the shoulders and arms. Raise the arms over the head. Often the writer becomes engrossed in the task at hand, losing all sense of time and bodily discomforts. When in the "zone," the writer may ignore warning signs or the little discomforts that she knows will lead to trouble. This is the equivalent of the athlete "playing in pain," but it is a habit the writer must avoid.

- Doctor Emil Pascarelli, of Columbia Presbyterian East Side Medical Center, recommends the "elbow flap": Hold the arms away from the body at the shoulders and let the arms flap or fall several times to relax the shoulder muscles and prevent static tension and fatigue caused by needlessly holding the arms away from the sides.

- The "wrist flop," gently shaking the arms to let wrists and hands fall loosely, also helps relax the muscles of the shoulders and forearms. At rest, assume a more comfortable posture and positioning of the arms and shoulders.

- Use a timer to remind you to take breaks, stretch, and change postures, or install a computer program that automatically prompts the writer to stop and do his exercises. Such a program reminds the writer to be careful, to interrupt his work and take a break, change position, and do some exercises.

You are an athlete! Prepare to work as an athlete prepares to compete. Warm up the shoulder muscles, and stretch, just like a sprinter or a linebacker or a baseball pitcher. Get ready to play. Get ready to write. Stretch and relax and move and change posture, just like the world-class athlete. Treat yourself accordingly!

For the computer worker, even the choice of recreation becomes important. For most, enough exercise to maintain conditioning is desirable, but the writer may need to avoid sports or games that require throwing and racquets, and impact sports that might add troubles to the shoulder. Just as a musician cares for the hands and arms, so must the writer. Equally important, limit sedentary activities such as watching movies or television or attending concerts. These contribute to adverse postures and static loading of the muscles and tendons of the arms and shoulders, aggravating the writer's upper-extremity problems. Remember that the arms and shoulders are vulnerable during recreation as well as work.

TREATMENT

Once the shoulder has been injured, the writer must be very careful: Treatment often requires care by a physician and a therapist knowledgeable about the problems of computer workers.

Gradual conditioning and stretching must be performed within the tolerance of pain. Avoid the fallacy that "if it hurts it must be doing some good," and live as pain-free as possible.

There is no substitute for resting the affected parts, which for the writer is the entire body. In the absence of a specific and speedy remedy, once symptoms arise, the writer must take into account any daily activities that cause fatigue, static loading of muscles, and mental exhaustion. Healing occurs during periods of rest and sleep, and it cannot occur during periods of activity similar to those that caused the injury in the first place.

Treatment begins with awareness of the importance of proper positioning at the computer and posture of the shoulders: Shoulders should be back and down. Use heat and/or ice on sore and painful areas, accompanied by gentle massage of the muscles. Massage may be accomplished in several ways in addition to the usual manual massage. Skin-fold massage of sensitive areas of the shoulders can be done by the writer at times, but the individual usually cannot reach all of the areas of the neck and shoulders that may need massage. Skin-fold massage may be done by a cooperative spouse or friend.

Squeezing a rubber ball has *no* place whatsoever in the treatment of any disorder of the computer worker (in fact, squeezing adds to muscular tightness and strain), but lying on the floor on a small rubber ball or tennis ball and rolling back and forth as a type of massage to the upper back and shoulders can be done by the individual when no other option is available. The writer may find this form of massage painful until he can moderate the amount of pressure placed on the rubber ball. Periods of massage should be brief: a minute or so.

Relaxation techniques (which will be discussed further in chapter 14) aid in reducing tension of the shoulder muscles. General physical conditioning, such as walking, swimming, or other exercise that does not add more stress and fatigue to the shoulders, assists in reducing tension of the shoulders.

Seeking the care of a knowledgeable physician and experienced physical therapist in the problems of the writer may be needed. Occasional injection of a local anesthetic or cortisone into tender bursa areas, or certain (but not all) tendon areas, and tender muscles near the shoulders may help. These areas often become less tender and painful with time and through the use of therapeutic exercises and stretches, without the need for other interventions.

On occasion, a mild analgesic medicine gives some comfort, but, as was mentioned previously, pain medicine must not under any circumstances be used to allow the writer to continue to abuse the muscles of the upper extremities.

To avoid mouse-shoulder syndrome (which was detailed earlier in this chapter) move the mouse toward the center of the work space. Directly in front of the writer is desirable but usually impractical. Use a curved finger posture as recommended for the keyboard and operate the mouse with the tips of the fingers, not with the finger pads or with the finger straight. Use two fingers—the index and the middle finger—on the mouse button if at all possible. This reduces the static tension and extension posture which occurs when using only the index finger on the mouse.

Above all, avoid reaching to the side for the mouse and holding the arm away from the body for extended periods. Move the mouse more centrally even if you must move the keyboard somewhat to the side. A small board extending off the edge of the table or desk and clamped in place allows the mouse to be operated without reaching to the side. The writer merely rotates the arm at the shoulder with no added effort or static loading. Usually, the mouse is placed on a pad lower than the keyboard, which makes the position of the shoulder awkward and strained. Raise the mouse pad to the level of the top of the keyboard.

12

The Neck:
"Up in the Withers"

"Let the galled jade wince, our withers are un-
wrung."

William Shakespeare, *Hamlet*

Writers and computer workers often complain of
stiffness and tightness of the muscles of the back of
the neck and across the top of the shoulders on first
arising in the morning and after long periods of sitting at the computer keyboard. Muscle tightness of
the neck produces complaints that extend far from
the neck itself. Headache, burning sensations over
the scalp, soreness toward the shoulder blades, and a
feeling of light-headedness may be associated with
muscle tightness of the neck, since how we perceive
ourselves in space depends in part on the tone of the
muscles of the neck and lower spine. A feeling of fatigue and a weak sensation of the neck and shoulder
muscles which the writer may not associate with

long sessions of writing may occur. Although a slight "grinding" sensation with movements of the neck is normal, this sensation may be more intense and frequent with tightness of the neck muscles.

FINDINGS ON EXAMINATION

A physical examination may reveal a limited range of motion of the neck, especially when tilting the head to the side. This is due to tightness of the postural muscles of the neck. Diffuse tenderness of the neck muscles or the appearance of tender nodules in the muscle called "fibrositic nodules," especially at the base of the skull, mid-way down the neck, and toward the upper angle of the shoulder blade, are common. Often, skin-fold tenderness of the neck occurs, which may be manifest as a severe burning pain when the skin of the neck is lifted or twisted. Under normal circumstances, this lifting, twisting, or rolling of the skin produces no pain or discomfort.

On testing strength, the muscles of the neck and shoulders may be weak or have poor endurance.

CRS has some common features with other musculoskeletal disorders, such as fibromyalgia. Fibrositis and fibromyalgia are the most common names of a disorder characterized by muscle stiffness and pain in the neck, shoulders, and upper arms. Symptoms also include fatigue and tender points in specific areas. These tender spots or bands of muscle (the fibrositic nodules) occur at sites that are consistent from patient to patient. Although fibromyalgia can occur at any age, including childhood, it is most common between the ages of twenty and fifty. Most sufferers experience difficulty getting to sleep and/or wake without feeling rested. Fatigue tends to be present all day and not relieved by sleep.

The pain of fibrositis varies: aching, burning, deep, sharp or dull, needlelike, tingling, numbing, or cramping sensations. Usually, symptoms must be present for three months or longer before it can be considered fibrositis because many similar complaints which subside in a few days or weeks involve similar symptoms. Fibrositis tends to occur in those who are perfectionists, sensitive to demands made of themselves and others, who repeatedly evaluate the consequences of their actions, and those who have an acute awareness of body sensations.

CAUSE

Neck pain and soreness in the computer worker is usually due to sustained poor posture, causing static loading of the neck muscles. An ancient form of torture consisted of forcing the head to be held in a forward flexed position for extremely long times, during which the neck would become exquisitely painful. When finally allowed to raise his head, the victim experienced excruciating pain. Sitting for long hours at the computer or other activities where the head and shoulders are held forward and immobile are equivalent to this form of torture.

Emotional tension, deadlines, distractions, and other pressures tend to make the muscles of the neck and shoulders become tense in a defensive posture, as if preparing for an attack. Being "up in the withers," like a dog or cat with the fur on the back of its neck up, prepares the writer for the classic flight-or-fight reaction. Poor posture at the computer—chin jutting forward, rounded shoulders, shortening of the muscles at the front of the neck, and body hunched forward—greatly increases the risk of neck and shoulder pain and affects all parts of the upper extremities.

Chronic neck pain, often associated with migraine headaches, may be caused by the daily use of common, over-the-counter medicines, including aspirin, antihistamines, pseudoephedrine, ibuprofen, narcotics including codeine and hydrocodone, caffeine, some tranquilizers, barbiturates, nasal decongestants, and muscle relaxants. These medicines are often taken to treat the symptoms of headache and neck pain, but are short acting, so that the patient is in a recurring state of withdrawal. The symptoms of withdrawal from the medicines prompt the patient to take more medicine, creating a cycle of pain. Improvement occurs in 60 percent of individuals if these medicines are completely discontinued for at least three months.

PREVENTION

Awareness of the risks of poor posture and abnormal positions of the arms and shoulders is one of the biggest steps toward preventing injury. Proper posture with "head back, chin down" and "chin tucks" (an exercise described in chapter 15) reduces the postural demands of the neck muscles. The keyboard, monitor, and reference materials must be reasonably placed so that a neutral trunk posture is possible. If reference materials are in an awkward position, such as far to one side, comfortable posture is impossible. A proper chair with a high back, no arm rests, a forward tilt of the seat, and set at the correct height can make the difference between comfort and safety or pain and misery. If the writer uses the telephone extensively, an *effective* cradle for the handset or a headset preserves the posture of the neck and shoulders, reducing the likelihood of further wear and tear on the neck. For those who use the telephone frequently and for long periods, a headset prevents prolonged static loading of the neck muscles.

The muscles of the neck are especially susceptible to tension in the writer's life. Efforts to relax the muscles of the neck can include a change of scenery, walking, a massage, deep breathing with the diaphragm and abdomen, or taking a warm bath or shower. You are not alone in the matter of emotional and muscle tension. A multitude of techniques and methods to aid relaxation have been developed by psychologists. Volumes have been produced on the subject. Visit the local bookstore or library and find a method of relaxation that suits you best.

The subject of relaxation is covered in more detail in chapter 14.

Correct prescription lenses and glasses that fit properly will help prevent leaning forward and craning the neck, putting added static load on the neck muscles. Avoid a position in which the elbows are held akimbo. This creates all sorts of stress and muscle fatigue of the neck, shoulder, and arms and can cause damage to the wrists and hands.

Stretch the muscles of the neck, shoulders, pectorals, and jaw. Be gentle, but persistent. A "comfortably uncomfortable" pulling sensation that is not overly vigorous is desired. Hold the position for ten seconds. Stretching is often best done initially under the supervision of an experienced physical therapist.

Lighting makes an important difference to most writers. If the light is low or glaring, an inordinate amount of effort is required to write, putting strain on the postural muscles of the neck and shoulders as well as the eyes.

Good ventilation helps. In spite of the macho image of the writer surrounded by dense swirls of cigarette smoke in a cloudy, dark room, fresh air picks up the spirits as well as freshening the mind.

Excessive noise or distracting sound may be filtered out through concentration, but this takes its toll on the writer's energy and increases muscle tension in the neck. Focusing attention in the face of distractions becomes increasingly difficult and increases energy demands, especially as the writer ages. Strive to create an environment that will allow ease of concentration as much as possible. A little background noise may actually help, but the writer must be alert to when the noise becomes distracting.

Resolve personal conflicts, which is easier said than done, but anything that can be controlled to your advantage ought to be controlled. Sometimes decisions must be made; delaying decisions can prolong agony and increase muscle tension of the neck, shoulders, and arms, draining energy from the writer's task.

Even in the best of circumstances, the writer must work to maintain concentration to stay in the "zone" where he or she is productive. If these lapses of common sense are permitted by the writer, it likely will be expressed in tension of the muscles of the neck and shoulders. Rarely does a writer achieve the author's nirvana, what Herman Melville called "the calm, the coolness, the silent grass-growing mood in which a man *ought* always to compose."[1] Do the best you can to control circumstances.

TREATMENT

Once the neck becomes painful, achieving relief is no small task and the sooner it is attended to the better. If the muscles of the neck become tight and uncomfortable, the writer will probably continue to have some discomfort most of the time. In fact, mild discomfort, fatigue, heaviness, or soreness of the neck is an almost uniform manifestation of the modern human condition whether one is a writer or not. The use of local heat or ice to the neck, or heat and cold applications alternately, may greatly lessen muscle soreness and pain. Massage of the sore muscles of the neck and tender fibrositic nodules, especially skin-fold massage, can be carried out by an experienced therapist, but can be performed effectively by a spouse or friend with instruction.

Gentle range-of-motion exercises, stretching, strengthening, conditioning exercises, and other therapeutic exercises are detailed in chapter 15. If the writer or computer worker is having more than minimal discomfort, appropriate and judicious exercises are best carried out under the supervision of a skilled physical therapist after a thorough evaluation.

A special neck or *cervical pillow* used at night often provides additional relief of discomfort in the neck because the neck is particularly susceptible to abnormal postures during sleep. A bath towel can be rolled into an oval and placed under the neck in conjunction with a standard pillow to prevent the neck from assuming an awkward or forced posture during the night. Do *not* sleep prone on the abdomen, as this causes the neck to be placed in forced rotation. Other extreme postures of the neck and shoulders during sleep add to the discomfort of the muscles and joints that are responsible for maintaining stability of the neck.

Relaxation of the muscles of the neck, spine, and shoulders in combination with proper posture maintain the health of the neck muscles and reduce muscle tightness and pain. The correct posture is assumed by "head back, chin down, trunk straight" while standing, walking, sitting, and even sleeping.

Achievement of a good posture and keeping the neck in a pain-relieving position is not a small project. Learn and learn again to change position, move, stretch, and relax the postural muscles. Put this into practice day after day. Slouching at the keyboard seems to be favored by many students and writers, but it greatly increases the risk of injury to the arms, shoulders, back, and neck.

For some writers and computer workers, a period of time off work long enough to allow the muscles to recover may be the only solution. And when the writer returns to work, she must not fall back into old, injurious habits, but incorporate changes that will reduce the risk of more trouble with the neck and shoulders.

Local anesthetic or cortisone injections into trigger points of the neck muscles is occasionally warranted if pain persists. Usually, with re-education and maintaining good work habits, injections are not necessary. If all other measures fail and the writer is still experiencing difficulties, injection can give a great deal of relief. No guidelines can predict whether an injection will provide long-lasting relief or transient benefit, but the chances for relief improve with proper posture.

The neck is subject to many hazards, and often calls for specialized examination and treatment by a physician. In addition, specialized physical therapy may be required to evaluate and treat diagnosed conditions. The anatomical complexities of the neck do not permit a generic, definitive treatment without an examination by a physician, although most who experience difficulties such as muscle tension symptoms of the neck are able to carry on with their careers by making suitable modifications. The writer can never return to the prior abusive, injurious habits, but persistence and consistency with appropriate exercises and proper technique maximize the writer's chances for recovery.

NOTE

1. Herman Melville, Letter to Nathaniel Hawthorne, June 1?, 1851, in *The Melville Log,* 2 vols, by Jay Leyda, p. 412 (New York: Gordian Press, 1969).

13

The TMJ:
The Temporomandibular Joint

"But first he chewed grain and licorice, To smellen sweete."
Geoffrey Chaucer, "The Miller's Tale,"
The Canterbury Tales

The motions of the temporomandibular joint (TMJ), or the jaw joint, are complex; the joint glides, slides, and hinges. The cartilage of the temporomandibular joint is not as resistant or resilient to wear and tear as cartilage in most other joints. The joint may click or jump while eating or talking, and if damage is severe, it may lock or result in limited motion and ability to open the mouth. Complaints of gritting and grinding the teeth (bruxism), which may be unconscious, warn of difficulty.

Sleep is the most troublesome time when bruxism occurs. The writer may not be aware he grinds his teeth unless alerted to the fact by another. The writer may awaken in the morning with soreness of the muscle area in front of the ear (the masseter muscle), headache, or pain in the temporomandibular joint. As the problem progresses, pain and muscle tension involve other muscle groups, such as the muscles of the back of the neck and the trapezius muscles of the shoulders. Pain may even be felt into the front of the chest, raising the question of more urgent causes of chest pain.

FINDINGS ON EXAMINATION

Findings of tenderness of the TMJ (by palpating in front of the ear) and clicking or uncoordinated movements with a zigzag motion on opening and closing the jaw point toward problems with the temporomandibular joint. Trigger points in the masseter muscle of the face are occasionally so tender that these points require injection of a local anesthetic and cortisone.

CAUSE

Most problems with the TMJ are due to poor neck posture accompanied by clenching and grinding the teeth while at work or asleep. Eating French bread crusts, nuts, tough meat, hard candy, apples, etc. puts great pressure and loading stress on the soft cartilage of the temporomandibular joint. Tension and concentration increase the likelihood of clenching unconsciously. Even touching the upper and lower teeth together without clenching is enough to add considerable pressure to the joint because of the anatomy of the jaw and the temporomandibular joint. Even while driving or at the movies, many people unconsciously hold their jaw tightly clamped, adding to the static loading stress on the TMJ. Nevertheless, bruxism during the night is the most common cause of temporomandibular joint problems.

PREVENTION

Prevention requires being aware that the jaw joint can cause or contribute to neck and upper-extremity problems. Avoid gritting, clenching, and grinding the teeth together. Problems of the temporomandibular joint can be serious and should not be taken lightly.

TREATMENT

Treatment begins with the counsel, "lips together, teeth apart," an admonition given by dentists. This position takes the loading pressure off of the temporomandibular joint. Touching the tip of the tongue to the roof of the mouth while writing or driving or at other vulnerable times cuts down on the writer's ability to clench his teeth. Most of the treatment of problems of the TMJ are up to the individual to carry out:

- In front of a mirror, practice opening and closing the mouth slowly. Make the jaw open and close in a straight line, as this improves the mechanics of the temporomandibular joint and lessens pain and the tendency to brux.

- Apply moist heat or ice to the area of the TMJ and the masseter muscles. This reduces tightness of the muscle and inflammation of the temporomandibular joint.

- Gently massage the masseter muscle and trigger points in the muscle to reduce muscle soreness.

- Rest the temporomandibular joint by avoiding eating nuts, French bread crusts, or other foods that are hard to chew. Also avoid unnecessary chewing of gum, candy, and the like.

- Cut down on unnecessary talking (which may be a hardship for some).

- Take small bites of food that are easy to chew without forcibly clenching the teeth.

- Practice relaxation techniques aimed at treatment of the temporomandibular joint. Be aware of tension in the masseter muscles of the jaw. (These may be held tense even when not chewing or when the teeth are not clenched.)

- Adjust posture to a neutral spine position and shoulder position. This decreases stress and tension of the neck and jaw muscles.

Specialized treatment by a dentist and physical therapist skilled in the care of TMJ disorders is frequently required to control problems of the temporomandibular joint. Often a "night guard" or a soft cap over the upper teeth, such as those worn by basketball players, is created to keep the teeth partially separated even if bruxism occurs. The night guard decreases mechanical pressure on the surfaces of the temporomandibular joint and is often effective in reducing pain in those who cannot otherwise control bruxing at night. In severe problems with the temporomandibular joint, a special, hard dental splint is worn day and night.

Although the temporomandibular joint seems far removed from the writer's hands and arms, it may be the source of much difficulty, and if the temporomandibular joint is not attended to, all other efforts to control problems with the upper extremity in the computer worker may fail.

14

Relaxation Techniques and Other Preventive Measures

RELAXATION TECHNIQUES

"Rest is the sauce of labor."
Plutarch, *Moralia*

Relaxation exercises help relieve the stress-tension cycle. One can relax by tensing and releasing muscle groups, through a passive activity such as meditation, or through activities such as hiking and swimming. Other relaxation procedures, such as recalling pleasant personal images, breathing exercises, and cognitive cue-controlling procedures, are also used. Relaxation is as much a state of mind as a physical state. It is an acquired skill; suddenly acquiring the ability to relax is not likely, but gradual improvement occurs over a period of time.

Transcendental meditation has become a well-known method of achieving a state of relaxation over the past several decades. Transcendental meditation centers on posture, breathing rhythmically, and the individual's mantra, a simple word or monotonous sound.

Dr. Herbert Benson writes in *The Relaxation Response* that the opposite of the "stress response," what he terms the "relaxation response," occurs naturally.[1] Benson has developed a relaxation method that involves the major points of formal meditation. His method requires the following:

- A quiet environment with as few distractions as possible.

- A "mental device" repeated over and over which helps to focus thoughts and prevents the mind from wandering, such as the "monosyllabic, non-emotion-arousing word *one*. Any single syllable which you do not mentally associate with anything else will work as well." The mental device is the equivalent of the mantra of meditation.

- A passive attitude, not worrying about distracting thoughts, but focusing on the simple, monosyllabic sound.

- A comfortable position that avoids undue muscular strain; not lying down but sitting in some comfortable posture.

Once a comfortable position has been found, sit quietly, unmoving, with eyes closed to eliminate visual distractions. Relax all the muscles. Begin at the feet and progress to the face. Concentrate on each part as it is relaxed. Breathe through the nose, saying the word "one" or a similar word.

This should be continued for fifteen to twenty minutes. After this time, sit quietly for a few minutes before opening eyes, then stay in the same position for a few minutes with the eyes open.

A deep sensation of relaxation may not be achieved initially. Practice twice a day, but not within two hours of a meal because digestion inhibits mental relaxation.

Simpler methods, such as deep breathing exercises, may also be beneficial for relaxation: Lie on the floor with a small pillow under the head. Knees should be bent so that both feet rest comfortably flat on the floor about a foot apart. Place one hand on the chest and one hand on the abdomen. Inhale through the nose, taking deep breaths with diaphragmatic breathing. Exhale through the mouth whispering "aaaaaah" with jaw relaxed.

Another method of relaxation involves "convincing" yourself that you are relaxed. First, close your eyes. Then, say to yourself, "I am relaxed. I am quiet." Then, shift your focus to individual parts of your body, saying things like, "My right arm is heavy, my left arm is heavy. My right leg is warm and relaxed, my left leg is warm and relaxed." Once you can feel a body part relax, move on to the next, finally ending with phrases like, "My body is warm and relaxed. I am at peace. My mind is at rest."

Another approach involves deliberately tensing muscle groups for thirty seconds (until some discomfort is experienced), then releasing them. Wait sixty seconds, then tense another muscle group. The preliminary exertion aids in relaxation. After some experience the writer becomes more aware of what a tensed muscle feels like.[2]

A similar method of relaxation which involves alternately tensing and relaxing groups of muscles, aids in learning relaxation as well as increases awareness of states of body tension:

First, sit as comfortably as possible (do not cross the legs). Take a deep breath, and let it out slowly. Tell yourself to relax. Then, bend the arms at the elbows, make a firm fist with both hands, and bend the wrist downward while tensing the muscles of the upper arm to produce a sense of tension (but no pain) in the hands, forearms, and upper arms. Hold this position for five seconds, then slowly let the tension out halfway while concentrating on the sensations in your arms and fingers as the tension decreases. Hold the half-tension for five seconds, then slowly let the muscle tension out the rest of the way and rest the arms in the lap. Concentrate on the difference between the tension and the relaxation (which increases through voluntary relaxation over an additional ten to fifteen seconds). Breathe normally, concentrate on the muscles, and give yourself the mental command to relax with each exhalation. Repeat this for seven to ten breaths.

Repeat the sequence by tensing the calf and thigh muscles by straightening out your legs while at the same time pointing your toes downward. Hold the tension for five seconds, then slowly relax the tension out halfway and hold for five seconds before slowly relaxing entirely.

Cross the palms of the hands in front of the chest and press them together to tense the chest and shoulder muscles. At the same time, tense the stomach muscles. Follow tensing of muscles by partial relaxation and breathing as above.

Arch the back and push the shoulders back as far as possible to tense the muscles of the upper and lower back, being careful not to tense the muscles too much. Repeat the same procedure of slowly releasing the tension halfway, hold, then release fully, and complete with the breathing exercise and the mental command as the back muscles are relaxed.

Tense the neck and jaw muscles by thrusting your jaw outward and drawing the corners of your mouth back. Release the tension slowly halfway, hold, and relax fully. Let your head droop into a comfortable position and let the jaw slacken while concentrating on those muscles and breathing.

Wrinkle the forehead and scalp to tense those muscles, hold for five seconds, relax halfway, then fully. Focus on relaxing the facial and scalp muscles completely, use breathing and the command to "relax" to deepen relaxation.

Further relaxation may be achieved while sitting in a relaxed position, taking a series of short inhalations (about one per second), until the chest is filled and tense, holding for five seconds, then exhaling slowly while telling yourself to relax. Repeat three times. Concentrate on breathing comfortably, using the abdomen more than the chest. Deepen relaxation while exhaling. Abdominal breathing is more relaxing than chest breathing and reduces tension of the neck muscles.[3]

When under stress, monitor areas of tension in order to relax those areas in particular. Repeat breathing relaxation whenever you have the opportunity. This will help to control emotional arousal in stressful situations.

Not all of these steps may be appropriate to relaxation during writing, but they may be useful afterward to allow the writer to "decompress" and to get a good night's sleep rather than continue to be troubled by creative tensions. After discovering which muscle groups are the most tense, select exercises to reduce tension in those particular muscles. These exercises can also be performed intermittently at the keyboard.

Imagery or fantasizing about peace and tranquility (a calm and peaceful scene, a deserted beach, a field of flowers, a quiet night, etc.) is another method that has been recommended to achieve a state of relaxation. Imagine being a flower, a leaf floating in the wind, etc., in an effort to let muscular tension go.

Oriental methods of muscular and mental relaxation have found favor in the West, especially tai chi, a method of slow, rhythmic movement that provides some conditioning as well as relaxation. A number of relaxation audio- and videotapes that have aided some individuals to improve their ability to relax are available. For some people, prayer may be the most effective method of reducing stress and obtaining a state of relaxation.

OTHER PREVENTIVE MEASURES

"Although the world is full of suffering, it is full also of the overcoming of it."

Helen Keller, *Optimism*

We live in a culture that honors our athletes for giving 110 percent and playing in pain, risking permanent injury. More important to the "athletic" nature of writing is learning to live as pain-free as possible. That means preparing the work area to reduce the likelihood of injury; warming up and cooling down; and keeping the arm, hand, and shoulder muscles in proper condition. After being away from writing for a period of time, the writer ought not try to write all day any more than a sensible baseball pitcher would try to pitch a complete game when not in physical condition after a long winter's layoff.

Be aware of and pay attention to early symptoms: muscle tightness, limited motions of the wrists and shoulders, swelling of the hands and forearm muscles, and numbness or tingling of the arms or hands. The key to continue writing and the use of the keyboard is early detection and prompt treatment. The longer a writer has been injured, the longer it takes to recover. While no definite duration of symptoms has been shown to lead to permanent disability of the writer, those who have continued to work at the keyboard for months or years after the first sign of trouble may have great difficulty in recovering from their injuries. These people often require a period of time off nearly twice as long as the amount of time that they experienced symptoms. And a small number never recover.

Writers are advised to take measures to make certain that they do not injure themselves and impair their ability to do what they do: write. Take periodic breaks, move about, get out of the chair, plan ahead.

The limitations placed on writers by computer-related syndrome mainly result from stiffness and pain. Static loading of the musculotendinous unit must be relieved and prevented as much as possible—any posture or attitude that results in prolonged static loading puts the writer at risk for injury. In addition, repeated grasping and twisting are especially hazardous. Temper cold and uncomfortable surroundings as much as possible and wear clothing suitable to keep the extremities warm.

In order for the writer to minimize the chances of injury these general measures should be taken into account:

Posture, both while writing and while away from writing, including while resting and sleeping, is of paramount importance to the writer. Maintaining correct posture is a constant struggle, because the act of writing at the keyboard seems to invite bad habits (slumping or slouching, propping the feet up on a stool, craning the neck).

Breaks are necessary to relieve static loading of the postural muscles and their tendinous attachments. Regular breaks of at least five minutes per hour may not be enough for many people, but a brief rest every fifteen minutes or so may suffice.

Change positions frequently. When our mothers admonished us to sit still, we sat still. Today's mothers may well advise their computer-literate children to move, sway, and change position, and *not* to sit still. Stand up. Raise arms overhead and wiggle the fingers. Stretch the muscles of the forearms, shoulders, and neck. Additionally, when our mothers said, "Sit up straight!" they were right, and that is apt advice for computer keyboard workers of today.

Pay attention to the chair and the workstation, making sure that is not too efficient, that it encourages and requires the writer to move about. Simple changes that are effective in reducing the risk of injury can usually be made.

Use heat to warm the hands and forearms before starting to write, and a combination of heat and ice after writing or during breaks, to lessen swelling of soft tissues of the arms and hands and reduce pain and stiffness.

Gently massage the hands and forearm muscles as well as the neck and shoulder muscles between periods of writing to aid in maintaining comfort.

Wearing gloves at night, such as cotton jersey gardening gloves, keeps the hands warmer and thus improves circulation, although soft, slightly elastic gloves may reduce swelling.

Avoid clenching the hands at any time, especially at night. Find a sleeping position that ensures that the hands are in a neutral position.

Be aware of risks involved in commuting for those who must hold on to a railing or steering wheel, or carry a heavy briefcase or luggage. Planning and lightening the load while using proper body mechanics can help. Even a backpack adds to the workload of the shoulders and neck. Keeping the load small and reasonably light, whether in a briefcase or backpack, is common sense. For some, a waist pack may be useful. Be aware that driving may cause tension and fatigue of the very muscles the writer must conserve. Holding the arms and shoulders frozen at the steering wheel with little movement while driving is as stressful as it is at the keyboard. Tight spots in traffic often unconsciously cause the driver/writer to grip the steering wheel with all of their might.

Keep a realistic outlook. The hands can do only so much before they rebel in pain, tightness, and swelling.

Maintain general physical conditioning, such as walking or swimming, without putting the arms and hands through even more physical abuse. Writing, though an athletic performance by the hands and forearms, is not aerobic activity for the heart and lungs. This includes maintaining a healthy, balanced diet and weight control. Obesity and an enlarged girth cause the arms to be carried away from the sides of the chest and contribute to hazardous hand positions.

Take vacations. A change of environment may do wonders if writing has stalled or the arms become weary.

Be sure to care for the eyes. Strive for adequate lighting, elimination of glare and reflection, properly fitted glasses, and a screen with a large enough font to eliminate leaning forward to read. Perform range-of-motion movements of the eyes, from side to side, near to far, up and down, to break the static position of the eyes. Placing reference materials on a stand near the mid-line of the dominant eye reduces the effort of eyes, neck, and shoulders. Further, head position and posture of the upper back is largely determined by the direction of the visual target.

Treat your fingers, hands, and arms like a sensible athlete would and avoid injury by over-use.

Avoid rings, bracelets, and other jewelry. They are additional hazards to anyone who works with their hands because they may get caught on a nail or hook, increasing the risk of serious injury.

Use assistive devices around the home, such as milk carton holders, key holders, car door openers, and jar openers. Many simple, inexpensive aids may be purchased through occupational therapists, physical therapists, medical supply stores, or most office equipment stores.

Use the proper method and tools when writing longhand. One of the most neglected aspects of the writer's tools is the pen or pencil. Most people use narrow, hard-to-grip pens and pencils that put enormous stress on the joints, muscles, and tendons of the fingers, hands, and forearm. A large-barrel pen or an adapter, found in office supply stores, that enlarges the diameter of the pen or pencil is a simple device that reduces this common and unnecessary stress to the hands and forearms. Instead of using only the wrist and hand to write, move the arm from the shoulders and avoid cramped wrist postures as the pen crosses the page from left to right.

Periodically reassess your career. The writer, like everyone, must balance material benefits of the rat race against personal needs and satisfactions. Speed, work output, and the need to continue writing must be weighed against the risk of serious injury and loss of livelihood. Speed is the demon for many writers, while we must recall that nearly all of the great masterpieces were written with a quill or a dip ink pen. Even the typewriter has produced little of sustained value, and the computer even less. Nonetheless, the computer has many advantages, but speed kills!

NOTES

1. Herbert Benson, *The Relaxation Response* (New York: Morrow, 1975).

2. Michael C. Matteson and John M. Ivancevich, *Managing Job Stress and Health* (New York: Free Press, 1982).

3. Frank L. Smoll, Ph.D., and Ronald E. Smith, Ph.D., "Psychology of the Young Athlete: Stress-Related Maladies and Remedial Approaches," *Pediatric Clinics of North America* 37 (1990): 1021–46.

15

The Exercises

"The wise for cure on exercise depend."
John Dryden

Many exercises may be used to reduce the risk of computer keyboard injury. The exercises suggested here are a concise program that can be performed with minimal equipment in a reasonably brief period of time, and cover the most common areas needing intervention.

Almost every computer worker needs to improve in several or all of the following areas:

- Strength and endurance of the muscles that move and stabilize the shoulder blades.

- Abdominal muscle strength and endurance in a functional, neutral spine position.

- Flexibility of the neck muscles, especially those on the sides of the neck (the scalene muscles), which flex the neck to the sides.

- Flexibility of the muscles of the front of the chest (the pectoral muscles).

- Flexibility of the forearm muscles.

- Strength and endurance of the weight-bearing quadriceps muscles of the thighs.

- Flexibility of the muscles of the hands.

- Endurance of the eye muscles.

Regular exercise does not have to be strenuous to be beneficial. Slow, steady progress is the key to success for any exercise program, which requires gradual but important life changes for the computer worker. Walking is an excellent exercise when done regularly. A home exercise program is nearly always necessary and often crucial to prevent injury. Goals must be objective and measurable, but formal testing is not necessary. If the computer worker is self-employed, self-monitoring is essential.

The writer must be willing to participate in an exercise program regularly to gain maximum benefit. The goals are to achieve maximum *comfort,* to achieve maximum *efficiency* while working or writing, and to *avoid injury* while maintaining reasonable productivity. It is important to remember the following points for the program to be effective:

- Maintain normal spinal curves with support of the back in a properly adjusted, comfortable chair.

- Efficiently distribute the forces of gravity over the entire musculoskeletal support system.

- Maintain neutral shoulder position.

- Maintain comfortable, functional forearm, wrist, and finger position.

- Maintain enough adjustability to allow a variety of supported positions and movement options without sacrificing health, efficiency, or productivity.

Prior to beginning to work or write the writer should check his posture and the seat height, angle, and depth. The hip joints should be slightly above the knee joints. Place the feet flat on the floor with some weight on the feet.

The head and neck are aligned in a neutral position relative to the rest of the spine, with the preservation of the normal spinal curves without muscle strain.

Bring the shoulders up, back, and down until they are in a neutral position. The shoulder blades ought to be resting comfortably on your rib cage with the neck muscles relaxed.

Make sure the wrists are relatively neutral and forearm, wrist, and hand muscles relaxed.

EXERCISES BEFORE STARTING TO WRITE*

1. Neck Stretches

- While looking straight ahead, bend the ear toward the shoulder until a stretch is felt on the opposite side of the neck, hold for fifteen seconds. Repeat on the other side.

- Side bend as above and rotate the head until a stretch is felt on the opposite side, hold for fifteen seconds. Repeat on the other side.

- Bend chin forward toward the chest until a stretch is felt along the back of the neck. Hold for fifteen seconds.

- Bend forward until a stretch is felt, add rotation to the right and then left, hold for fifteen seconds each side.

- Use diaphragmatic breathing while stretching in order to gradually increase the range of motion.

2. Shoulder Repositioning

- Bring shoulders up as high as you can, then back as far as possible, and then down as low as they can get on the ribs.

- Relax the shoulders.

---

*These exercises should also be performed intermittently while at the keyboard (every thirty minutes or so).

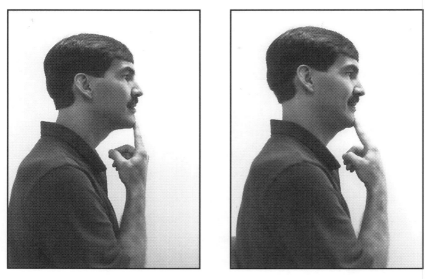

"Chin tuck" by moving the chin back slightly to improve neck posture and reduce tension of the scalene muscles of the neck. This facilitates better posture of the shoulders, which are rotated back and down through the shoulder repositioning exercise.

- Repeat frequently, at least every fifteen to twenty minutes.

3. Chin Tucks

- Slide the chin back toward the neck with a scooping motion of the head, as if someone were pulling a string attached to the back of the head.

- Then relax. Do not push the chin forward.

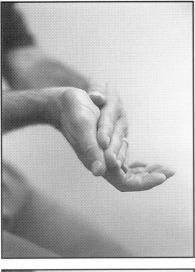

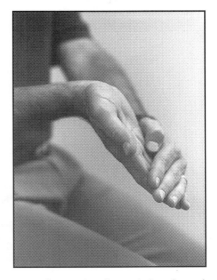

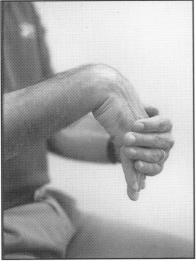

a. Stretch the right hand with gentle, sustained pressure in the palm by the left hand, hold for ten to fifteen seconds.

b. Stretch the right hand and forearm muscles with gentle, sustained pressure on the fingers of the right hand by the left hand.

c. Stretch the extensor muscles of the right forearm with gentle, sustained pressure on the back of the hand by the left hand.

Repeat all steps for the other hand.

4. Diaphragmatic Breathing

- Breathe deeply and slowly, letting the abdomen move forward while inhaling, and back while exhaling.

- Avoid excessive use of the neck and chest muscles and do not let the shoulders rise with breathing.

- Repeat frequently. Even ten breaths can make a difference.

5. Wrist and Finger Stretches

- With the palm up and the elbow bent to 90 degrees, use the opposite hand to gently pull the wrist and hand down and back toward the body. Slowly and gently progress down toward the fingertips to gradually increase the intensity of the stretch. One may feel a stretching sensation, but *do not* use pressure that causes pain. Hold for fifteen seconds.

- Repeat procedure with palm down.

- Repeat with the elbow straight out in front of the body and palm facing up.

- Repeat with palm down.

6. Arm, Wrist, Hand Shaking; The "Wrist Flop"

- With palms up, sideways, and down, gently oscillate the arms at the shoulders at a comfortable rate.

- Emphasize relaxing the neck, shoulders, and arms.

- Eliminate all unnecessary muscular activity.

HOME EXERCISE PROGRAM

In addition to the exercises that the writer performs at his computer workstation, a home exercise program is essential to maximize the benefit to be gained from proper conditioning and posture awareness. Such a program will also increase skill in relaxation techniques. Very little space and equipment is required for this home exercise program.

1. Side-Lying Arm Circles

- Lying on one side with the spine straight, hips and knees bent to 90 degrees, and head positioned on a pillow in line with the spine, place the "bottom hand" on the "top knee."

- Extend "top hand" at shoulder height with the palm down, and *slowly* move the hand up toward the head, tracing a large circle around the body. Keep the elbow relatively straight, and keep the hand as close to the floor as possible without pain or straining. If too much sensation of stretching, pain, or other discomfort occurs, raise the hand away from the floor to a more comfortable level.

- Continue as long as relaxation and gentle stretching of the shoulder and pectoral muscles occurs. Usually ten repetitions is enough.

- Caution. Do not perform this exercise if you have had a shoulder injury or you cannot perform this exercise without pain.

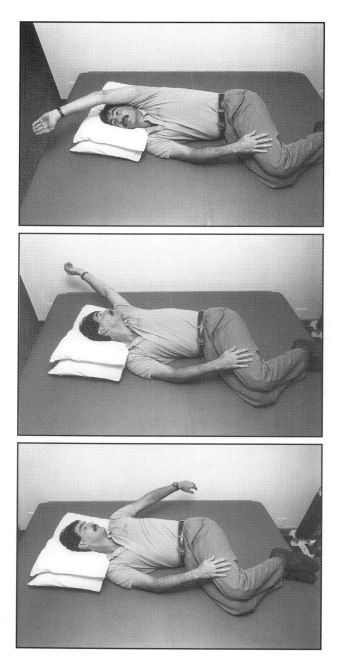

Side-lying arm circles, done slowly to stretch the shoulder muscles, especially the pectoral muscles of the front of the chest.

2. Scapular Endurance Prone

- Lying on the stomach with a large pillow or exercise ball under the abdomen, pull the shoulder blades back and down to their lowest point.

- Keeping the elbows straight, hold the arms by the sides of the legs.

- Maintaining this shoulder blade position, lift the arms even with the mid-line of your body, approximately three inches off the ground.

- Do not allow the shoulder blades to creep up toward the ears or to slide out to the side of the rib cage.

- Gradually increase the amount of time of holding the arms raised against gravity in this position to two minutes.

- Repeat with the arms overhead, and with the arms at 45 degrees and at 90 degrees from the sides of the body.

3. Side-to-Side Rolling

- This exercise requires the use of a four- or six-inch diameter ETHAFOAM® roll.*

---

*ETHAFOAM® is a polyethylene foam normally used for packing created by the Dow Chemical Company. It is often used by physical therapists as an exercise tool. Some physical therapy supply companies stock the rolls, or they can be ordered from Optimal Performance Physical Therapy, 1923 Oak Park Boulevard, Pleasant Hill, California 94523.

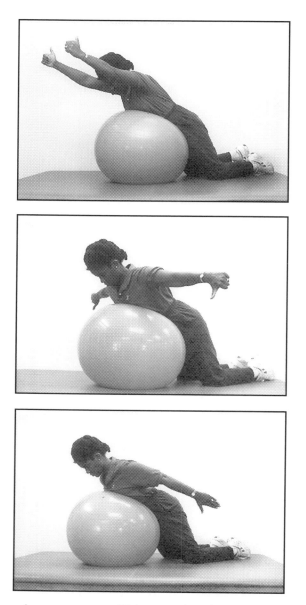

Scapular endurance prone. This exercise strengthens the trapezi-us muscles of the upper back and neck. A stool or chair can be substituted for the therapy ball. Gradually increase the time of holding each position to two minutes.

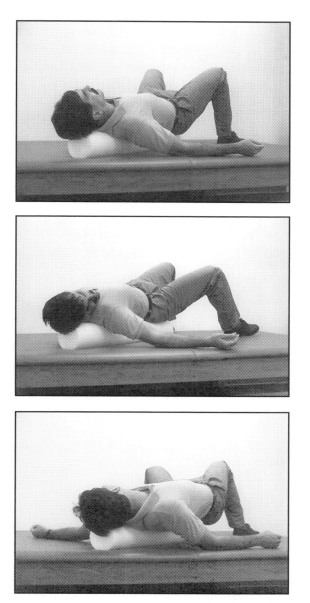

Side-to-side rolling on an ETHAFOAM® roll. The shoulders and hips are rolled in a horizontal plane. The head rolls to the opposite side. This exercise massages and relaxes the shoulder, back, and neck muscles.

- Recline with the spine, head, and tailbone on the foam roll.

- Position the feet approximately shoulder-width or slightly wider apart. Use the legs to control movement of the body to slowly roll from side to side.

- Keep the pelvis level, without letting it roll over the side of the foam roll.

- Allow the head to slowly roll to the opposite side from the pelvis at the same rate as the trunk and pelvis are rolled to the side.

- Repeat ten times to each side, or as desired for comfort.

- Do not use the ETHAFOAM® roll exercise in the presence of back pain or other medical conditions unless approved by your physician or physical therapist. Muscular soreness often occurs after rolling, especially the first time, but usually subsides after the first few occasions of performing the foam roll exercise. Do not continue to use the roller if muscle soreness persists.

4. Supine Marching

- Lying on the back with knees bent and feet flat on the floor, gently roll the pelvis forward and backward through pain-free range of motion only.

- Stop mid-way in the movement of the pelvis and tighten the stomach muscles as in a cough.

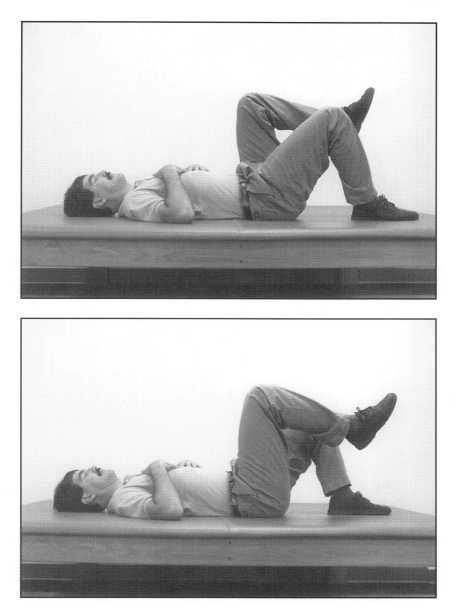

Supine marching. As one knee is flexed, the other is partially straightened as if walking. The lumbar spine is to be held in a neutral position. Continue as long as the curve of the lumbar spine can be held flat in a neutral position. Work up to three minutes. This exercise strengthens the thigh, abdominal, and back muscles.

- Keep the abdominal muscles tight enough to lift one leg up to a 90-degree angle without moving your back. Hold the position.

- Without letting the back move, lift the other leg as the first leg is lowered to the floor, and continue "marching," keeping the back immobile. Gradually work up to three minutes of marching. Stop if you experience symptoms of pain or fatigue, or if you cannot hold the back immobile.

5. Linebackers

- Standing with feet shoulder-width apart, position the spine in neutral, keeping the back straight.

- Bend at the hips, knees, and ankles until the elbows can be rested on the thighs. If unable to bend this far, start with hands on the knees and gradually work to a deeper squatting position.

- Keeping the back straight throughout, slowly bend and almost straighten the knees.

- Continue until fatigued or unable to keep the back straight.

- Gradually progress until the exercise can be sustained continuously for three minutes with the back straight.

Do not continue this exercise if pain occurs in the knees, back, or anywhere else. Some muscular soreness in the thigh muscles (quadriceps muscles) is to

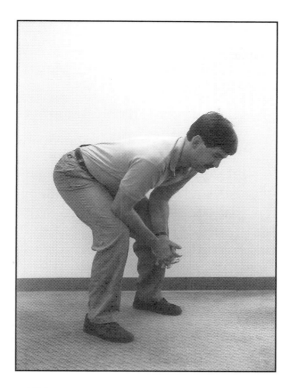

Linebackers. This exercise strengthens the thigh (quadriceps) and abdominal muscles. Progress to holding the position for three minutes.

be expected at first, and can be relieved by gently stretching the sore muscles (bend the knees until a stretch is felt in the front of the thighs; hold for thirty seconds). Do not overdo this or any other exercise.

Be aware of the "symptom threshold," and recall that once it is surpassed, the possibility and/or extent of injuries greatly increases. The following is a list of *warning signs*. If any of these occur, stop the activity or keyboard use and consult your physical therapist or physician:

- Pain.

- Numbness.

- Tingling of the arms or hands.

- Coldness or paleness of the fingers and hands.

- Aching which does not resolve quickly upon changing position.

- Swelling.

- Loss of sensation or an abnormal sensation in the hand or other body area.

- Dizziness or lightheadedness.

- Nausea.

- Difficulty focusing the eyes.

- Difficulty maintaining concentration.

- Any symptom that increases in frequency, intensity, or duration.

Most of these symptoms will subside after a short rest period, a change of position, or a change in activity. However, they may be warning signs of a problem such as tendinitis, bursitis, repetitive strain injury, or any other form of CRS. If left untreated, minor problems may become major ones. Early intervention is essential.

16

Life after CRS

RETURNING TO WRITING

"Now thou art gone and must never return."
John Milton, "Lycidas"

After a period off work due to computer-related syndrome, the writer must take a cue from the athlete returning after a long layoff: most athletes require six weeks to return to anywhere close to their desired performance level. Returning to writing is the same. It takes time, and can't be rushed. Build tolerance for writing a little at a time, but always stop before the onset of pain or other discomforts.

Warm-up and cool-down become even more important after an injury. Take frequent breaks sufficient to allow the muscles and soft tissues to recover. Move and change position to avoid static loading.

Above all, avoid old habits. Work within your pain-free ability, even if it is only a fraction of the time you formerly worked. Don't be stubborn or proud. Your goal is to return to work and writing safely and comfortably, not to prove yourself. Resist doing the same thing to your upper extremities a second time.

Use a mirror to monitor hand position. In this way, old awkward positions and injurious habits can be identified and avoided. Occasionally look down at your hands while you write. They are your bread and butter.

Take short relaxation breaks during periods of writing even if you don't feel the need for it at the time. Monitor your posture frequently. Sit straight, feet flat on the floor, and take deep, relaxing breaths from the diaphragm.

Change goals from production output to writing pain-free. Rock back in your chair, look out the window. Get a drink of water, but not from a glass or carafe at your side. Go to another room or out in the hall and get it at the water fountain. If necessary, learn two-finger typing for at least some keyboard use. Some old detective and sports writers wrote great volumes with two fingers. It sacrifices speed, but increases movement of the arms and shoulders.

Special keyboards may be helpful for some, but keyboard design is not the entire solution. If the writer continues to use bad habits, new computer keyboard design will not help. The keyboard angle, height, size (distance between the keys), resistance forces, and cushioning of the bottoming of the keys play important parts. Keyboards that allow angling or tilting of the keys have a place in special circumstances.

The Dvorak or American Simplified Key System designed in the 1930s greatly reduces the traffic of the fingers along the keyboard by placing the most commonly used letters along the middle row of keys. It is easy to use, but allows increased speed and the problems that increased speed may cause. This keyboard arrangement may be beneficial for those with CRS symptoms of the fingers and forearms, but it tends to increase static loading positions of the arms and shoulders by reducing movement. Those who choose to use the Dvorak system for the fingers must pay attention to the need to move the arms and shoulders.

New and special equipment, such as scanners to copy large amounts of print in a short time with little keyboard input, may reduce some writing demands. Voice recognition and voice-activated computer programs and equipment may be of use to those who are severely limited. Other innovations will surely be developed by injured workers and those whose needs require them to change their ways.

FAILURE TO RETURN TO WRITING

> "Pleasure is oft a visitant; but pain
> Clings cruelly to us."
> John Keats, "Endymion"

The incidence of those who cannot return to writing or keyboard use is small, but 1 or 2 percent of injured writers are not able to return to work even after an absence of as long as three years.[1]

Injured writers or workers must seek professional help: a physician knowledgeable about work-related problems of the upper extremity, a physical therapist with special training or experience with computer workers, or an occupational therapist who specializes in hand therapy. A social worker sympathetic to the needs of keyboard workers and occasionally a psychologist or psychiatrist can be of great assistance in particularly difficult circumstances encountered by injured workers.

The writer must be willing to accept the existence of the problems related to keyboard use, to take the responsibility for making changes, and to work with physicians and therapists toward recovery. Avoid becoming the "help-rejecting-complainer" who scuttles all efforts of assistance. In the best of circumstances, treating a severely injured writer is a demanding, difficult, and often frustrating undertaking for the medical professional as well as for the writer.

In rare instances, pain becomes intractable and no longer follows the normal pathways, evolving into a new entity—chronic pain. At this point, efforts to reverse or remove the cause of the pain are abandoned and extensive efforts to control pain must be undertaken. Special pain clinics at some university medical centers and private clinics have developed for those who might require care and treatment for this most difficult problem.

THE FUTURE

"The future is bound to be a bright, useful one."
Dwight D. Eisenhower, 1960 speech

Writers' careers today largely depend on their ability to use the computer keyboard effectively and safely. Businesses and business schools are beginning to recognize that their future depends on the health of their computer keyboard workers. Although some companies and managers wish to deny the magnitude of the problem, estimates of the number of people suffering from CRS range as high as 25 percent.[2] Many companies are now taking steps to insure their future by instituting prevention of CRS and insisting on early treatment. Forward-looking companies have established exercise rooms where employees can go to perform exercises specifically designed to help prevent the problems of the keyboard worker. Writers who write at home can do the same with little expense. The discipline to do the exercises regularly and to adopt optimal postures and techniques at the keyboard resides with the individual. A program can be installed in the computer that will prompt the writer to stop writing, and then list specific exercises and stretches to be done.

Children and teenagers are also at risk. They start to use wrist rests early, and most slump in their chairs or assume other postures that are likely to cause disorders of the upper extremities. Intent on their homework or video games, hazardous positions and postures become habitual and difficult to change.

Research programs dealing with the problems of the keyboard worker and writer are underway and making some progress, but progress is slow and expensive. Industry and government sponsor programs, but the problem is enormous. The modern writer and computer worker must take advantage of what is available now, such as adjustable-height workstations and comfortable-touch keyboards.

If the evolutionists are right, future generations will develop muscles of the hand and forearm that will evolve to be like the hummingbird's wings—able to make one hundred or more keystrokes per second. At an average of eight keystrokes per word, that's twelve words per second, 720 words per minute, 43,200 words per hour, or 345,600 words, or a good-sized novel, in an eight-hour day. *War and Peace* in a day and a half. Until such evolution has occurred, however, slow down. Even hummingbirds take periodic rests. Take care of your hands, arms, neck, and shoulders. Use good posture and proper technique. Remember, writers are armchair athletes who need to take care of their physical assets.

Stay updated. More information that will be important to the writer will come in the years ahead.

NOTES

1. Michael L. Adams, "Outcome of Carpal Tunnel Surgery in Washington State Workers' Compensation," *American Journal of Industrial Medicine* 25 (1994): 527–36.

2. David Rempel, "Overview of Upper Extremity Musculoskeletal Disorders: Epidemiology and Risk Factors," paper presented at the conference for Occupational Ergonomics: Control of Work-Related Upper Limb Disorders, Sacramento, California, April 10–12, 1996.

Appendix

Where to Get Help

Not all physicians or even orthopedic surgeons are interested or skilled in the care of the soft tissue disorders or upper-extremity musculo-skeletal disorders of the computer worker. But many hand surgeons; some rheumatologists and physiatrists (specialists in physical medicine or rehabilitation); and certain physical, occupational, and hand therapists are well trained and interested in occupational disorders of the upper extremity. A few special ergonomic clinics (which focus on the "biotechnology" of the health of the workplace and tend to be located in larger population areas) may be consulted. A few large medical centers provide clinics for the medical problems of musicians, which are very similar to those of the writer.

The following are organizations and publications dedicated to the problems of the writer and computer worker:

The National RSI Foundation
220 S. Desplaines Avenue
Chicago, IL 60661

The VDT News: The Computer Health & Safety Report
Box 1799
Grand Central Station
New York, NY 10163

Some helpful books include the following*:

Stephanie Brown. *The Hand Book*. New York: Ergonome, 1993.

Kate Montgomery. *Carpal Tunnel Syndrome: Prevention and Treatment,* 3d ed. San Diego: Sports Touch, 1994.

Paul Davidson. *Chronic Muscle Pain Syndrome,* rev. ed. New York: Berkeley Books, 1996.

Emil Pascarelli and Deborah Quilter. *Repetitive Strain Injury: A Computer User's Guide.* New York: John Wiley & Sons, 1994.

---

*Although quite a few books are available, there are not many we would be willing to recommend. That so few good ones are available was one of the motivations for writing this book.

WORKSTATION AND POSTURE CHECK LIST

Sit with feet flat on floor, some weight on the feet.

Hips slightly higher than knees.

Neutral spine and neck posture.

Shoulders down and back.

Chin tuck.

Elbows held loosely against the sides of the chest.

No forearm rests.

Wrists even with or slightly lower than elbows.

Wrists straight or slightly drooped.

No wrist rests.

Wrists canted slightly outward.

Relaxed, curved fingers.

Type with the tips of the fingers.

Frequent changes of position of the hands, arms, and trunk.

WORKSTATION EXERCISES

(Before writing and intermittently while writing)

1. Neck stretches
2. Shoulder repositioning
3. Chin tucks
4. Diaphragmatic breathing
5. Wrist and finger stretches
6. Arm, wrist, and hand shaking
7. The "wrist flop"
8. The "elbow flap"

DAILY HOME EXERCISES

1. Side-lying arm circles
2. Scapular endurance prone
3. Side-to-side rolling
4. Supine marching
5. Linebackers